The Effective Prevention and Management of Systemic Fungal Infection

Second edition

Titles of related interest in the UK Key Advances in Clinical Practice Series

SOLID TUMOURS

The Effective Management of Breast Cancer, 1st, 2nd and 3rd edns

The Effective Management of Colorectal Cancer, 1st, 2nd, 3rd and 4th edns

The Effective Management of Lung Cancer, 1st, 2nd and 3rd edns

The Effective Management of Malignant Melanoma

The Effective Management of Ovarian Cancer, 1st, 2nd and 3rd edns

The Effective Management of Prostatic Cancer

The Effective Management of Renal Cell Carcinoma

The Effective Management of Urological Malignancies

HAEMATOLOGICAL MALIGNANCIES

The Effective Management of Non-Hodgkin's Lymphoma, 1st and 2nd edns

The Effective Prevention and Management of Systemic Fungal Infection in Haematological Malignancy, 1st and 2nd edns

The Effective Prevention and Management of Common Complications of Induction Chemotherapy in Haematological Malignancy

The Effective Management of Chronic Lymphocytic Leukaemia

SYMPTOM CONTROL

The Effective Management of Cancer Pain, 1st and 2nd edns

The Effective Prevention and Control of Symptoms in Cancer

The Effective Prevention and Management of Post-Operative Nausea & Vomiting, 1st and 2nd edns

HEALTH POLICY

NICE, CHI and the NHS Reforms: Enabling excellence or imposing control?

Clinical Governance and the NHS Reforms: Enabling excellence or imposing control?

Managed Care Networks: Principles and practice

The Effective Prevention and Management of Systemic Fungal Infection

Second edition

Edited by

Archie Prentice FRCPath
Consultant Haematologist, Derriford Hospital, Plymouth, and President, British Society for Haematology

Tom Rogers MA MSc FRCPath FRCPI
Professor of Clinical Microbiology, Imperial College, Faculty of Medicine, Hammersmith Hospital, and Past Chairman, Antifungal Working Party of the British Society for Antimicrobial Chemotherapy

Andrew Miles MSc MPhil PhD
Professor of Public Health Sciences, and Editor in Chief, Journal of Evaluation in Clinical Practice, Barts and The London, Queen Mary's School of Medicine and Dentistry, University of London, UK

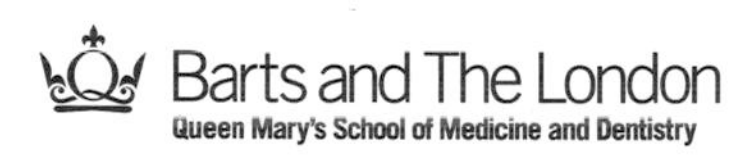

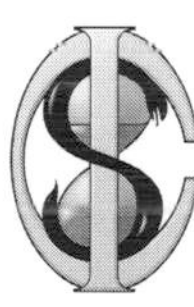

Intensive Care Society

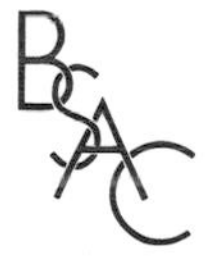

British Society for Antimicrobial Chemotherapy

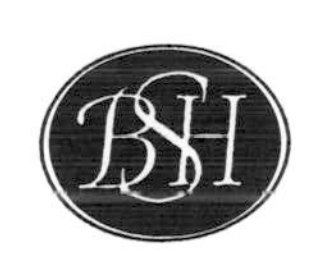

British Society for Haematology

AESCULAPIUS MEDICAL PRESS
LONDON SAN FRANCISCO SYDNEY

Published by

Aesculapius Medical Press (London, San Francisco, Sydney)
PO Box LB48, London EC1A 1LB, UK

First published 2004

British Library Cataloguing in Publication Data
A CIP catalogue record for this book is available from the British Library

ISBN: 1 903044 34 0

Further copies of this volume are available from:

Claudio Melchiorri
Aesculapius Medical Press
PO Box LB48, Mount Pleasant Mail Centre, Farringdon Road, London EC1A 1LB, UK

Fax: 020 8525 8661
Email: claudio@keyadvances4.demon.co.uk

Copy edited by The Clyvedon Press, Cardiff, UK

Typeset, printed and bound in Britain
Peter Powell Origination & Print Limited

Contents

Contributors

Rosemary A Barnes MB BS MA MSc MD MRCP FRCPath, Consultant Medical Microbiologist and Senior Lecturer in Medical Microbiology, University Hospital of Wales, Cardiff

Richard Barton PhD, Clinical Scientist, Mycology Reference Centre, Leeds General Infirmary and University of Leeds, UK

Nicole MA Blijlevens MD, Consultant Haematologist, Department of Haematology, University Medical Centre St. Radboud, Nijmegen, The Netherlands

James P Burnie MA MSc MD PhD DSc MRCP FRCPath, Professor of Medical Microbiology, Manchester Royal Infirmary and University of Manchester, UK

Christopher Dalley MD MRCP MRCPath, Specialist Registrar in Haematology, Royal London Hospital, UK

J Peter Donnelly PhD, Co-ordinator for Supportive Care Studies, University Medical Center St Radboud, Nijmegen, The Netherlands

A Glasmacher MD PhD, Attending Physician in Haemato-oncology, Department of Internal Medicine, University of Bonn, Germany

Rick Keays MD FRCP FRCA, Consultant in Intensive Care Medicine, Chelsea and Westminster Hospital, London, UK

Chris Kibbler MA FRCP FRCPath, Consultant Medical Microbiologist, The Royal Free Hospital, London, UK

NVS Kumar MRCP, Specialist Registrar in Haematology, Derriford Hospital, Plymouth, UK

Elizabeth M Johnson BSc PhD SRCS, Consultant Mycologist, and Head, Mycology Reference Laboratory, Health Protection Agency, Bristol, UK

Adrian Newland MA FRCP FRCPath, Professor of Haematology, St Bartholomew's and the Royal London School of Medicine, Royal London Hospital, London, UK

Archie G Prentice MB FRCPath, Consultant Haematologist, Derriford Hospital, Plymouth, UK

Malcolm Richardson PhD FIBiol FRCPath, Associate Professor of Medical Mycology, Haartman Institute, University of Helsinki, Finland

Tom Rogers MA MSc FRCPath FRCPI, Professor of Clinical Microbiology, Imperial College Faculty of Medicine, Hammersmith Hospital, London, UK, and Past Chairman, Antifungal Working Party of the British Society for Antimicrobial Chemotherapy

Simon AJ Rule BM BS BMedSci MPhil MRCP FRCPA, Consultant Haematologist, Derriford Hospital, Plymouth, UK

Neil Soni MD FRCA, Consultant Anaesthetist, Lead Clinician in Intensive Care Medicine, Chelsea and Westminster Hospital, London, UK

DL Turner BSc MRCP MRCPath, Consultant Haematologist, Torbay Hospital, UK

Preface

Much of current practice in managing systemic fungal infections, as Rogers points out within chapter 1 of this volume, is based on studies conducted over the past 20 years which have demonstrated a significant increase in incidence. For example, the National Nosocomial Infection Surveillance program in the USA reported a near doubling in incidence over the decade 1980–1990, which was largely attributable to *Candida* spp. In one large retrospective study of candidiasis, again conducted in the 1980s, the attributable mortality was 38%. More recent controlled clinical trials of antifungal therapy suggest that in non-neutropenic critical care patients the morbidity associated with candidaemia is lower than this figure but these are an important group in whom there is a greater awareness of the problem of systemic candidiasis. Aspergillosis is perceived to be the leading systemic mycosis in patients with haematological malignancy, especially those treated by allogeneic bone marrow or stem cell transplantation. The insensitivity of diagnostic investigations has prevented accurate incidence data from being obtained for this disease but in a recent German post mortem study invasive aspergillosis was reported to be the most frequent cause of death due to fungal infection and the main patient groups were those who shared profound neutropenia as a risk factor. Earlier, effective treatment of candidiasis has probably reduced mortality rates but has been associated with a shift in *Candida* species. Recent multi-centre and local surveillance studies show that *Candida albicans* accounts for no more than 50% of cases of candidiasis and correspondingly the proportion of infections due to non-*albicans Candida* spp., notably *Candida glabrata*, has increased; morbidity appears similar irrespective of the particular species involved.

The agents of nosocomial fungal infection are principally *Aspergillus* and *Candida* and many of the risk assessment techniques used to investigate microbiological hazards can be applied to opportunistic fungi, as Richardson discusses in chapter 2. Risk analysis is a structural approach to the reduction of risk which includes risk assessment, risk management, risk communication and risk monitoring. Risk assessment, for example, consists of four steps: hazard identification, exposure assessment, dose–response assessment and risk characterisation and involves the calculation of both the probability and impact of disease. The management of risk involves the examination of ways in which either the probability of disease or its severity can be reduced. Many of the environmental hazards contributing to invasive aspergillosis, for example, have now been identified, including unfiltered air, defects in hospital ventilation systems, food items and possibly hospital water supplies and stringent environmental controls in transplant units have included high efficiency air filtration, positive pressure ventilation and frequent room air changes. Although there have been several well-documented examples of aspergillosis outbreaks as a result of hospital demolition and reconstruction, it has not, as the author shows, always been possible to demonstrate elevated spore counts in clinical areas during building work and the possibility of community-acquired aspergillosis must be considered. These risks can usually be effectively minimised and very few studies have linked environmental exposure to cases of invasive aspergillosis. The exposure pathways for nosocomial yeast infections include carriage on healthcare workers' hands, contaminated surfaces and medical devices. The environment also may become contaminated with yeasts, but the relative importance of this reservoir remains unknown.

In chapter 3, Blijlevens and Donnelly continue the discourse on yeast infections. As the authors remind us, although neutropenia is known to be an important risk factor in cytotoxic treatment related infectious complications, the implications of damage to the epithelium of the intestinal tract have been largely ignored. Indeed, when combined with colonisation by *Candida*, mucosal barrier injury provides a portal of entry for the yeast. The authors discuss methods for determining changes in gut function such as impaired gut integrity and increased gut permeability and examine the relation between mucosal barrier injury and colonisation on the one hand and the onset of candidiasis on the other. This information can, as they make clear, be used to select patients at high risk for invasive disease which includes those treated for acute leukaemia with anthracyclines or high-dose cytarabine containing regimens as well as those receiving a haematopoietic stem cell transplant after total body irradiation. Such high-risk patients are the ones most likely to benefit from anti-fungal prophylaxis and who would normally not require any additional measures for prevention.

It is to a detailed consideration of the prophylaxis of systemic fungal infections to which we turn in chapters 4, 5 and 6. *Candida* infection, as Soni and Kibbler point out in chapter 4, is an acknowledged problem in the critically ill surgical patient. The group of patients that are at risk can be identified by known risk factors but there is little certainty of the incidence of confirmed *Candida* sepsis. Although increased surveillance would seem a logical endeavour in these patients the role of prophylaxis is, as the authors discuss, less easily defined. There are, of course, very limited data and such as there are suggest that although prophylaxis might be helpful in reducing colonisation and infection to a limited degree, it certainly does not prevent it completely. The benefits are therefore unclear and there may be negative aspects. Indeed, there is circumstantial evidence that prophylaxis may induce a change in flora and subsequently, when infection occurs, it might be with a more resistant *Candida* species. Moreover, prophylaxis, especially at low dosage, might jeopardise the value of surveillance and might diminish the likelihood of early detection of breakthrough infection. Additionally, prophylaxis at dosages that are subtherapeutic may not prevent infection and on a community or Unit level, a change in flora might expose other patients to increased risk. Given these considerations, Soni and Kibbler believe it would be hard to recommend prophylaxis on a widespread basis. They suggest a much more focused approach to identifying very high-risk populations, those with a high probability of infection and in these either a more aggressive approach to prophylaxis or an earlier treatment intervention that might in effect be the same end point.

To improve the efficacy of anti-fungal prophylaxis in neutropenic patients with haematological malignancies, many factors must be considered and it is to these that Turner, Glasmacher and Prentice turn in chapter 5. The authors emphasise that the incidence and antifungal drug susceptibility of individual organisms causing systemic fungal infections should be known in each institution/population but these data are rarely available, partly because diagnostic techniques are applied inconsistently across the UK. They recommend that the risk of infection with different levels of intensity of therapy should be assessed by prospective identification of each fungal infection encountered in individual protocols, followed by retrospective analysis. There has been, of course, some progress which suggests a spectrum from very low risk (e.g. conventional out-patient chemotherapy for lymphoma) to a very high risk (e.g. matched, unrelated allografts with severe GvHD). But prospective risk analysis is rarely tackled in randomised controlled trials of therapy for haematological malignancies mainly because of heterogeneity of effort in the diagnosis of systemic fungal infections. Effective targeting of SFI prophylaxis also requires, the authors emphasise, accurate assessment of the efficacy/toxicity of individual drugs. As they point out, there is an abundance of PK/PD data and RCT results for several drugs. But the development of these studies has been haphazard and the interpretation of their results hampered by a paucity of the data described above. Effective prophylaxis in patients with haematological malignancies requires *in vivo* activity against a wide range of fungi (particularly *Candida* and *Aspergillus*, exchangeable oral or i.v. delivery with equal systemic efficacy (to cope with gut "failure") and minimum toxicity. Few drugs have met these targets and currently there are only two available, itraconazole and voriconazole. The history of the development of the first suggests that we should now investigate the potential of the other in appropriate patients.

There has been, as Keays describes in chapter 6, a substantial increase in the incidence of fungal infection in the immunocompromised patient, whether that compromise is due to critical illness, human immunodeficiency virus (HIV) infection, solid organ transplant or haematological malignancy. Undoubtedly, broad spectrum antibiotic use has contributed to this problem but higher clinical suspicion, more acceptable antifungals and improvements in diagnosis have aided recognition of this apparent epidemic. The problem may be mitigated by sensible antimicrobial policies but it certainly appears here to stay, at least for the foreseeable future. The issue of prophylaxis against fungal infection has, Keays emphasises, to take account of the population of patients targeted. In liver transplant recipients, for example, survival is unquestionably improved by antifungal prophylaxis, but the evidence in other groups is either sparse or arguable. Whereas haematology patients have neutropenia that is likely to last a few weeks, HIV-infected patients have an immune compromise that can last for years. What is most desirable, the author feels, is to identify infection and treat it promptly, but therein lies the problem. Diagnosis is problematic and a delay in treatment can be life-threatening. Although anti-fungal prophylaxis does help with controlling the uncomfortable symptoms of mucocutaneous infection it is less effective in preventing systemic infection and may lead to emerging resistance. This produces a situation one does not want: a systemic fungal infection that is even more difficult to treat. As a policy, Keays therefore feels that prophylaxis may well be flawed.

It is to diagnosis of infection and to the issue of resistance to anti-fungal therapies that we have committed Part Three of the volume. In chapter 7, Barton considers that the role of improved laboratory diagnosis is to enable earlier identification and therefore more effective treatment of systemic fungal infections and to reduce unnecessary empirical therapy. As this author shows, radiological investigation (CT or MRI scanning) is of proven use particularly for the diagnosis of invasive aspergillosis, but has logistical limitations. Culture of blood or bronchoalveolar lavage, as alternative approaches, is relatively easy though known to lack sensitivity. Histological evidence of tissue invasion together with culture of biopsy material remain gold standard diagnostic criteria for invasive fungal infections, but such material is rarely available and so, for sensitive laboratory diagnosis, two approaches have emerged: antigen testing and DNA testing by PCR. The detection of serum galactomannan for the diagnosis of invasive aspergillosis uses a standardised commercial kit offering good values of sensitivity and specificity (>90%) and intra-laboratory reproducibility. Reports of PCR-based tests for fungal DNA proliferate in the literature and in some cases excellent results are reported for their use in diagnosing fungal infections. However, as the author describes, these are all "in house" tests and there are many variables (including specimen type, extraction methods and PCR product detection methods) that make comparisons between PCR tests or between DNA and galactomannan detection virtually impossible. In the few comparisons of PCR and serum galactomman tests in the diagnosis of invasive aspergillosis different conclusions have been obtained about the importance of molecular tests and their role in the management of patients at risk from systemic fungal infection. Thus the standardisation of molecular testing is an important priority in the advancement of the laboratory diagnosis of systemic fungal infections.

Until the late 1980s antifungal drug resistance was a rare phenomenon, limited to a few cases of resistance to amphotericin B and well-documented resistance to flucytosine. However, as is the case with antibacterial agents and as Johnson points out in chapter 8, the increasing use of antifungal agents has led to the selection and induction of resistant strains and contributed to a shift in the spectrum of organisms causing infection. Antifungal drug resistance has not so far proved to be as problematic as that experienced with antibacterial agents but, as she notes, both intrinsic and emergent resistance are encountered and antifungal susceptibility testing can help in the guidance of prescribing practices. Standardised methods for susceptibility testing of yeasts and moulds have been introduced and although there are still certain reservations over the test methods, their widespread application makes national and international comparisons of susceptibility trends possible. Emergent resistance in some yeast species, seen predominantly with flucytosine and fluconazole, has been linked, Johnson shows, to inappropriate prescribing practices for specific infections in certain patient groups while modification of treatment strategies and control of underlying disease have reduced the incidence of emergent resistance in recent years. Intrinsic resistance, which is generally consistent and predictable, is encountered in an increasing number of yeast and mould species as the spectrum of organisms causing invasive disease broadens. Elucidation of resistance mechanisms has helped to explain the evolution of resistance within a given isolate and in populations and may therefore, she feels, lead to the rational development of new broad-spectrum antifungal agents.

Part Four of the volume, in two chapters, provides a thorough review of the place of antifungal interventions in the management of invasive disease. In the first chapter, Donnelly, after reviewing the current prerequisites for an antifungal drug – that it can be given safely and effectively both orally and parenterally to provide broad spectrum activity against *Candida* species and the common moulds as part of prophylaxis and treatment – provides a thorough review of the place of novel anti-fungal drugs in current clinical practice. Fluconazole has set the standard, as the author reminds us, because it is relatively safe and well tolerated and can be given orally as well as parenterally providing the flexible administration necessary to manage key patient populations in and out of hospital and with or without mucositis or gastrointestinal disturbances, but it possesses a limited spectrum of activity. Itraconazole should, perhaps, have been the prototype azole because it possesses the broad spectrum of activity desired. However, its passage from the bench to the patient has been long and tortuous – absorption was erratic necessitating a detour through pharmaceutics until a suitable solution was identified that could be tried, tested and approved and the development of a parenteral form necessitated a protracted retreat back to the laboratory until an acceptable formulation was found that eventually gained its license for use. Other triazoles, as Donnelly discusses, have been developed with similar spectra of activity as itraconazole of which three are proceeding through the registration phases. Voriconazole a derivative of fluconazole, has been licensed in the UK. The drug can be administered orally and parenterally and is effective in treating aspergillosis. Randomised controlled trials of empirical and specific therapy are in progress and the drug compares favourably with amphotericin B and other licensed forms of the polyene and may prove more effective. No direct comparisons with itraconazole are planned but trials of prophylaxis are being considered. Ravuconazole, another derivative of fluconazole, is currently proceeding through phase II studies and although a parenteral form is being developed the drug is only available in oral form limiting the scope of clinical studies. Its long half-life means once-daily dosing will be recommended. Posaconazole is a close relative of itraconazole and seems destined to follow a similar course as the drug is only available orally and efforts to develop a parenteral form have floundered. Like ravuconazole, the drug need only be given once daily because of its long half-life but again the scope for clinical studies is limited. Studies of prophylaxis are underway but the results are not expected for some time yet.

One of the most interesting developments so far, as Donnelly observes, has been the discovery of glucan synthesis inhibitors, the candins, which have been likened to penicillin in so far as they inhibit the synthesis of the cell wall for which there is no counterpart in the human host. Consequently they are relatively well tolerated and should prove the safest of the antifungal agents. Caspofungin has a licence for salvage treatment of aspergillosis. The activity of this drug against *Candida* species is also good and phase III studies have been completed for treating candidiasis. Micafungin (FK-463) and anidulafungin (LY303366) are two other candins in the early stages of development possessing similar properties to caspofungin but are being investigated in the first instance for their efficacy in treating refractory candidiasis. The principal weakness of the candins is the lack of an oral form and to overcome this they will most likely be employed in the same way as amphotercin B and its lipid formulations, namely, for empirical, pre-emptive and specific therapy. One of the triazoles will probably be used for primary prophylaxis and follow-up or maintenance therapy (also referred to as secondary prophylaxis) the most likely candidates being posaconazole or ravuconazole assuming both overcome the many obstacles such drugs face in the long haul to registration.

Standard approaches to the management of systemic fungal infection, as Barnes points out in chapter 10, are based on the use of amphotericin B imposed on a background of "protocol-driven" prophylaxis, empirical and pre-emptive antifungal therapies in patients considered at-risk. The continued rise in the incidence of infections and the considerable mortality in immunocompromised patients has led, as she notes, to a re-evaluation and the introduction of more aggressive treatments and immunocompromised patients with systemic infection may need a combination of fungicidal drugs, immunomodulation or surgery. The number of broad-spectrum antifungal agents available is, thankfully, increasing and lipid preparations of amphotericin, newer triazole agents, echinocandins, and potentially synergistic combinations incorporating flucytosine or terbinafine have been used successfully. However, not all drugs are, as Barnes points out, fungicidal against all species and the results of *in vitro* susceptibility testing do not always accurately reflect clinical outcome. Decisions must therefore be based on individual patients, infecting species and site of infection. Patients with systemic infection display marked immune dysfunction and in addition the immune response may be modulated by the fungus itself and at the level of the antigen presenting cell. Growth factors used both to increase phagocyte numbers and as immunomodulators are widely used but, as this author reminds us, our understanding of the mechanisms involved is limited and knowledge from animal models cannot necessarily be extrapolated to the human situation. Surgery has been recommended as adjuvant therapy particularly in aspergillosis and zygomycoses but intervention of this type has been limited by the concerns of high perioperative morbidity and mortality associated with the presence of neutropenia and thrombocytopenia in many of the patients involved. Recent reports have not, however, borne this out and surgery undoubtedly has a place in management with acceptable operative morbidity and improved survival rates. Aggressive combination regimens, then, are being used increasingly but Barnes is clear that few, if any, randomised trials have been conducted in this context and the evidentiary basis for combination therapy relies largely on comparison with historical controls and results must therefore be interpreted with this observation in mind.

Part Five of the volume, the penultimate section, has been dedicated to a review of economic evaluations of treatment options in the prevention and management of systemic fungal infection and to a classification and discussion of typical service deficiencies and common clinical errors in treatment. Economic evaluations of medicines, as Dalley and Newland point out in chapter 11 are, of course, now routinely done but no clear methodological standards have emerged by which comparisons may usefully be made. Although in general the direct acquisition costs of drugs are used, it is now clear that other indirect costs and benefits must be taken into consideration, some of which may not be easily attributable to healthcare resources. The impact on quality of life is crucial, as the authors emphasise, and this may vary from patient to patient depending on age and clinical circumstances. The rate of invasive fungal infection, as they observe, has doubled over the past two decades, reflecting more intensive chemotherapy, the increasing use of antibiotics, and a growing population at risk. Amphotericin B, the drug of choice, particularly in the neutropenic patient, is often considered inexpensive because of its low cost per vial but Dalley and Newland are clear that the frequency and cost of adverse reactions associated with amphotericin B may be high and must therefore be taken into account in any overall cost comparison.

The high incidence of proven invasive fungal infections in susceptible individuals at post-mortem serves to illustrate how common these problems are and how rarely they are diagnosed definitively and it is to issues such as these that Kumar and Rule turn in chapter 12. For the authors, it is important that patients at high risk of developing fungal infections are managed in a multi-disciplinary setting where there is firstly awareness of the potential for such infections and secondly an infrastructure that allows prompt diagnosis. This includes rapid availability of appropriate radiological and mycological investigation and finally appropriate and timely access to therapy. Ideally such patients, the authors advise, should be managed in a defined area with an appropriate environment to minimise exposure to such pathogens together with strict adherence to ward based hygiene. A robust algorithm for the management of high-risk patients should also be in place that is regularly audited and constantly reviewed in the light of changing epidemiological factors. Not all of these criteria are always met within hospitals and consequently it becomes possible to describe and classify common omissions, service deficiencies and sometimes frank error, as Kumar and Rule proceed to do.

Part Six of the text, the final part of the volume, provides an interesting overview of the place of immunological approaches in the management of systemic fungal infections and closes the volume with an exciting insight into yet another area of experimental therapeutics.

In the current age, where doctors and health professionals are increasingly overwhelmed by clinical information, we have aimed, in this Second Edition volume, to provide a fully current, fully referenced text which is as succinct as possible but as comprehensive as necessary. Consultants in Medical Microbiology, Haematology and Intensive Care Medicine and their trainees are likely to find it of particular use as part of their continuing professional development and specialist training respectively and we advance the volume explicitly as an excellent tool for these purposes. The book will also, we anticipate, function well as a reference volume for nurse specialists, hospital pharmacists and laboratory scientific and technical personnel and we commend the book to these colleagues for that purpose.

In conclusion we thank Gilead Pharmaceuticals Ltd for a grant of unrestricted educational sponsorship that helped organise a national symposium at The Royal College of Pathologists at which synopses of the constituent chapters of this volume were presented.

Archie Prentice FRCPath
Tom Rogers MA MSc FRCPath FRCPI
Andrew Miles MSc MPhil PhD

PART 1

Epidemiology and risk of SFI

Chapter 1

Epidemiological overview of morbidity and mortality from systemic fungal infection

Tom Rogers

Introduction

In the management of fungal infections, much of current practice is based on studies done over the past 20 years. These have consistently demonstrated a significant increase in incidence of invasive mycoses. For example the National Nosocomial Infection Surveillance Program in the USA reported a near doubling in incidence over the decade 1980–90 (Beck-Sague *et al.* 1993). This increase was largely attributable to *Candida* spp. In one large retrospective study of candidiasis, again done in the 1980s, the attributable mortality was 38% (Wey *et al.* 1988). Patients in this study had a wide variety of risk factors for infection. More recent controlled clinical trials of antifungal therapy suggest that in non-neutropenic critical-care patients the mortality due to candidaemia is substantially lower than this figure (Rex *et al.* 1994), but these are an important group in whom there is greater awareness of the problem of systemic candidiasis. Earlier and more effective treatment of candidiasis has probably reduced mortality rates but has also been associated with a shift in *Candida* species identified as pathogens. Multicentre and local surveillance studies show *C. albicans* accounts for no more than 50% of cases of candidiasis, and correspondingly the proportion of infections due to non-*albicans Candida* spp., notably *C. glabrata*, has increased (Pfaller *et al.* 2000).

Aspergillosis is perceived to be the leading systemic mycosis in patients with haematological malignancy, especially those treated by allogeneic bone marrow or peripheral stem cell transplantation. The insensitivity of current diagnostic investigations has prevented accurate incidence data from being obtained for this disease and undermined efforts to develop more appropriate preventative strategies (Prentice *et al.* 2000). However, in a recent German post-mortem study (Groll *et al.* 1996) invasive aspergillosis was documented to have significantly increased in incidence and had become the most frequent cause of death due to fungal infection in a University Hospital; the main patient groups shared profound neutropenia as the principal risk factor.

Candidiasis

Invasive candidiasis is often first manifested by invasion of the bloodstream, and in the USA, *Candida* spp. are reported to be the fourth commonest cause of bloodstream infection in the critically ill patient (Edmond *et al.* 1999). Surveillance studies of candidaemia have highlighted the changing epidemiology of *Candida* spp. Recently, the findings of the SENTRY study of *Candida* bloodstream infections done in North and South America, and Europe, between 1997–99 were reported. Data on 1184 episodes of candidaemia were collected (Pfaller *et al.* 2000). Overall, *Candida albicans* accounted for 55% of yeast blood stream infections (BSIs) but there were differences between continents. Whereas *C. albicans* caused 60% of BSI in Canada, 58% in Europe and 55% in the USA, the figure was 45% for Latin America. Of the non-*albicans Candida* species, *C. glabrata* was most common in the USA whereas *C. parapsilosis* was most common elsewhere.

To determine risk factors for development of candidaemia a prospective study was undertaken in six USA surgical intensive care units (ICUs) in the National Epidemiology of Mycosis Survey (NEMIS) (Blumberg *et al.* 2001). The incidence was 9.8 cases per 1000 admissions. Factors identified as being independently associated with increased risk of candidaemia were: prior surgery; acute renal failure; parenteral nutrition and, in post-surgical patients, presence of a triple lumen vascular catheter. Candidaemia was associated with a significantly increased mortality (41% with versus 8% without; $p < 0.001$) in this study. Perhaps surprisingly, prior colonization by *Candida*, as determined by rectal swab and urine cultures, was not associated with an increased risk of candidaemia. However, on the basis of molecular typing, patient-matched urine and blood isolates were typically indistinguishable, suggesting the urinary tract was an important source of the infection. Even though less than 50% were *C. albicans* most strains were sensitive to all antifungal drugs tested, including fluconazole. Similarly, susceptibility tests of *Candida* isolates from the SENTRY study showed these were mostly sensitive to all antifungals tested, including fluconazole (Pfaller *et al.* 2001).

Other studies in non-neutropenic patients have identified older age, hospitalisation in an ICU, retention of central lines and inadequate antifungal therapy as being significantly associated with a poor outcome (Luzzati *et al.* 2000).

In an earlier study of 106 patients with candidaemia from one centre an analysis was done of factors predicting mortality. A high APACHE II score, rapidly fatal illness, and sustained candidaemia were each independent predictors of mortality (Fraser *et al.* 1992). It is of interest that in the last patient group mortality was higher with non-*albicans Candida* spp. This issue was further analysed in a European Organisation for Research and Treatment of Cancer (EORTC) study (Viscoli *et al.* 1999). Whereas *C. albicans* accounted for 70% of episodes of candidaemia in patients with solid tumours, the corresponding figure for patients with haematological malignancy was only 36%. *Candida glabrata* was associated with a significantly poorer survival rate than other *Candida* species. Overall, crude mortality was 39% at 30 days post-candidaemia, candidaemia-associated mortality was 24%, whereas attributable mortality was 8%.

In a retrospective review of 139 patients with *C. glabrata* BSIs the most common admitting diagnosis was malignancy; however, prior abdominal surgery was strongly related both to development of the infection and subsequent mortality. Furthermore, the abdomen was most often documented as being the portal of entry (Gumbo *et al.* 1999). The hospital epidemiology of this organism is poorly understood but acquisition from environmental sources has been documented (Fidel *et al.* 1999).

Candidaemia significantly increases duration of hospitalisation, especially among elderly patients, and generates increased costs estimated in one USA study to be as high as $44,000 per case in 1996 (Rentz *et al.* 1998).

In a study of similar design to the earlier NEMIS study the incidence and risk factors for candidaemia on neonatal ICUs was investigated (Saiman *et al.* 2000). 1.2% of infants developed candidaemia with an incidence of 12.3 cases per 1000 discharges. Significant risk factors included: gestational age <32 weeks, 5 minute Apgar score of <5; shock and prior use of H2 receptor blockers. Although gastro-intestinal colonization was not shown to be a significant risk factor for development of candidaemia it was found to precede candidaemia in 43% of cases. This group also looked for risk factors for *Candida* colonization of neonates (Saiman *et al.* 2001). The use of third generation cephalosporins was associated with colonization by either *C. albicans* or *C. parapsilosis* whereas central venous catheters or intravenous lipid therapy were risk factors for *C. albicans*. H2 antagonists were a risk factor for *C. parapsilosis*. The incidence of hand carriage of *C. albicans* or *C. parapsilosis* by healthcare workers on these units was 5% and 19% respectively, prompting the authors to speculate that these represented an important source for acquisition by infants on neonatal ICUs.

Aspergillosis

The invasive form of this disease is widely reported to carry a mortality of >90%. Accurate data on incidence are difficult to obtain because of inadequate diagnostic methodology. In a prospective evaluation of a commercial *Aspergillus* antigen enzyme-linked immunosorbent assay (ELISA)-based detection test, 186 consecutive patients were studied (Maertens *et al.* 1999). The diagnosis of proven invasive aspergillosis (IA) required positive histology and culture. There were 27 cases of proven IA, giving an incidence of almost 15%.

Wald *et al.* (1997) have conducted probably the largest single-centre analysis of incidence, risk factors and morbidity from invasive aspergillosis in a bone marrow transplantation (BMT) patient population. There were 158 cases diagnosed from the records of 2496 patients. The occurrence of IA post-transplant had a bimodal distribution with peaks at 16 and 96 days. Significant risk factors for early cases included underlying disease, donor type, and transplant outside a protected environment whereas for the later cases the main additional risk factors were presence of graft-versus-host disease, neutropenia and steroid use. Perhaps surprisingly, only 30% of patients were neutropenic at the time of diagnosis. One-year survival for patients with IA was 7% compared with 54% for patients with no evidence of aspergillosis. As in this study, most cases are due to *A. fumigatus* but infections caused by currently less common *Aspergillus* species are increasing in incidence (Stevens *et al.* 2000). The fact that this species is present in the air in higher numbers compared with either non-*fumigatus Aspergillus* species, or other airborne fungal pathogens such as zygomycetes, may explain why it is a more frequent cause of pulmonary disease. Yet no specific virulence factors have been identified to explain how it causes disease in susceptible hosts (Latge 2001). Aqueous sources, such as hospital water tanks, have been suggested as a potential reservoir of pathogenic *Aspergillus* spp. (Anaissie *et al.* 2002). The epidemiological importance of this needs further study.

References

Anaissie EJ, Stratton SL, Dignani MC *et al.* (2002). Pathogenic *Aspergillus* species recovered from a hospital water system. A 3-year prospective study. *Clinical Infectious Diseases* **34**, 780–789.

Beck-Sague CM, Jarvis WR and the National Nosocomial Infections Surveillance System (1993). Secular trends in the epidemiology of nosocomial fungal infections in the United States, 1980–1990. *Journal of Infectious Diseases* **167**, 1247–1251.

Blumberg HM, Jarvis WR, Soucie JM *et al.* (2001). Risk factors for candidal bloodstream infections in surgical intensive care unit patients. The NEMIS prospective multicenter study. *Clinical Infectious Diseases* **33**, 177–186.

Edmond MB, Wallace SE, McClish DK *et al.* (1999). Nosocomial bloodstream infections in United States hospitals: a three year analysis. *Clinical Infectious Diseases* **29**, 239–244.

Fidel PL, Vazquez JA, Sobel JD (1999). *Candida glabrata.* Review of epidemiology, pathogenesis and clinical disease with comparison to *C. albicans. Clinical Microbiology Reviews* **12**, 80–96.

Fraser VJ, Jones M, Dunkel J *et al.* (1992). Candidemia in a tertiary care hospital. Epidemiology, risk factors and predictors of mortality. *Clinical Infectious Diseases* **15**, 414–421.

Groll AH, Shah PM, Mentzel C *et al.* (1996). Trends in the postmortem epidemiology of invasive fungal infections at a university hospital. *Journal of Infection* **33**, 23–32.

Gumbo T, Isada CM, Hall G, Karafa MT, Gordon SM (1999). *Candida glabrata* fungemia. *Medicine* **78**, 220–227.

Latge JP (2001). The pathobiology of *Aspergillus fumigatus. Trends in Microbiology* **9**, 382–389.

Luzzati R, Amalfitano G, Lazzarini L *et al.* (2000). Nosocomial candidemia in non-neutropenic patients at an Italian tertiary care hospital. *European Journal of Clinical Microbiology and Infectious Diseases* **19**, 602–607.

Maertens J, Verhaegen J, Demuynck H *et al.* (1999). Autopsy-controlled prospective evaluation of serial screening for circulating galactomannan by a sandwich enzyme-linked immunosorbent assay for haematological patients at risk for invasive aspergillosis. *Journal of Clinical Microbiology* **37**, 3223–3228.

Pfaller MA, Jones RN, Doern GV *et al.* (2000). Bloodstream infections due to *Candida* species. SENTRY Antimicrobial Surveillance Program in North America and Latin America, 1997–1998. *Antimicrobial Agents and Chemotherapy* **44**, 747–751.

Pfaller MA, Diekema DJ, Jones RN *et al.* (2001). International surveillance of blood stream infections due to *Candida* species. Frequency of occurrence and *in vitro* susceptibilities to fluconazole, ravuconazole, and voriconazole of isolates collected from 1997 through 1999 in the SENTRY Antimicrobial Surveillance Program. *Journal of Clinical Microbiology* **39**, 3254–3259.

Prentice HG, Kibbler CC, Prentice AG (2000). Towards a targeted, risk-based, antifungal strategy in neutropenic patients. *British Journal of Haematology* **110**, 273–284.

Rentz AM, Halpern MT, Bowden R (1998). The impact of candidemia on length of hospital stay, outcome and overall cost of illness. *Clinical Infectious Diseases* **27**, 781–788.

Rex JH, Bennett JE, Sugar AM *et al.* (1994). A randomised trial comparing fluconazole with amphotericin B for the treatment of candidemia in patients without neutropenia. *New England Journal of Medicine* **331**, 1325–1330.

Saiman L, Ludington E, Pfaller M *et al.* (2000). Risk factors for candidemia in Neonatal Intensive Care Unit patients. The National Epidemiology of Mycoses Survey study group. *Pediatric Infectious Diseases Journal* **19,** 319–324.

Saiman L, Ludington E, Dawson JD *et al.* (2001). Risk factors for *Candida* species colonization of neonatal intensive care unit patients. *Pediatric Infectious Diseases Journal* **20,** 1119–1124.

Stevens DA, Kan VL, Judson MA *et al.* (2000). Practice guidelines for diseases caused by *Aspergillus*. *Clinical Infectious Diseases* **30,** 696–709.

Viscoli C, Girmenia C, Marinus A *et al.* (1999). Candidemia in cancer patients. A prospective, multicenter surveillance study by the Invasive Fungal Infection Group (IFIG) of the European Organization for Research and Treatment of Cancer (EORTC). *Clinical Infectious Diseases* **28**, 1071–1079.

Wald A, Leisenring W, van Burik J-A, Bowden RA (1997). Epidemiology of *Aspergillus* infections in a large cohort of patients undergoing bone marrow transplantation. *Journal of Infectious Diseases* **175,** 1459–1466.

Wey SB, Mori M, Pfaller MA, Woolson RF, Wenzel RP (1988). Hospital-acquired candidemia. The attributable mortality and excess length of stay. *Archives of Internal Medicine* **148,** 2642–2645.

Chapter 2

The effective prevention of systemic fungal infection: precluding the risk of environmental exposure

Malcolm Richardson

Introduction

Nosocomial infection is defined as the acquisition of clinical infection as a result of medical intervention, and is usually applied to infections acquired in hospital. Examples include respiratory infection, such as pneumonia secondary to artificial ventilation, gastro-intestinal infection such as antibiotic-related colitis, intravenous-device related bacteraemia and post-surgical wound infections. The consequences of nosocomial infection range from simple colonisation, in which the infecting agent is present but is not causing clinical disease, to fulminant and life-threatening illness.

Despite the recent advances in diagnosis and treatment of invasive mycoses due to *Aspergillus* or other environmental fungi, these infections are always associated with a very high morbidity and mortality rate in patients at risk. Consequently, these diseases remain an increasing challenge during management of patients treated for leukaemia, recipients of allogenic stem cell transplants, and solid organ transplant patients.

Owing to almost constant need for updating and expanding of medical services, renovation and construction are common occurrences in healthcare facilities. Fungal spores are released during repair, maintenance and construction. The spores are small and stay airborne for considerable periods of time. They may also spread long distances. Exposure to fungal spores constitutes a very serious threat to immunocompromised patients. Water and moisture damage also occur often in hospitals. This may create fungal reservoirs that may lead to adverse health effects even among personnel. This review will focus on *Aspergillus* and aspergillosis. Background reading on the epidemiology of aspergillosis can be found in Manuel & Kibbler (1998), Ellis & Richardson (2000), Warnock *et al.* (2001), Richardson & Kokki (2002), and on the *Aspergillus* web site: www.aspergillus.man.ac.uk.

Aspergillus spores have caused much concern because they are ubiquitous, and invasive aspergillosis has a 75% fatality rate partly due to poor diagnostic methods (Richardson & Kokki 1998, 1999; Richardson & Ellis 2000). *Aspergillus* spore counts as low as 1–3 colony-forming units per cubic metre (cfu/m^3) have been found to cause infection. In addition, infection may occur because of colonisation, for example, of the paranasal sinuses, before hospital admission. Asthmatic patients and infants are also risk groups for fungal exposure.

Many of the risk-assessment techniques used to investigate microbiological hazards can be applied to opportunistic fungi. Risk analysis is a structured approach to the reduction of risk, which includes the risk assessment, risk management, risk communication and risk monitoring. Risk assessment consists of four steps: hazard identification, exposure assessment, dose–response assessment, and risk characterisation. This process involves the calculation of both the probability and impact of disease. The management of risk involves the examination of ways in which either the probability of disease or its severity can be reduced.

Many of the environmental hazards contributing to invasive aspergillosis have been identified, including unfiltered air, defects in hospital ventilation systems, food items, and possibly hospital water supplies. Stringent environmental controls in transplant units have included high-efficiency air filtration, positive-pressure ventilation and frequent room-air changes. Although there have been several well-documented examples of aspergillosis outbreaks as a result of hospital demolition and reconstruction, it has not always been possible to demonstrate elevated spore counts in clinical areas during building work. Furthermore, the possibility of community-acquired aspergillosis must be considered. These risks can usually be effectively minimized. However, very few studies have linked environmental exposure to cases of invasive aspergillosis.

The exposure pathways for nosocomial yeast infections include carriage on healthcare workers' hands, contaminated surfaces and medical devices. The environment also may become contaminated with yeasts, but the relative importance of this reservoir is unknown.

Finally, it must be stressed that nursing and medical staff should be educated in the special risks faced by the immunocompromised patient from the normal environment.

Prevention of aspergillosis

Prevention of aspergillosis is relatively difficult. Simple precautions – such as eliminating potted plants from patients' rooms and using barriers during hospital construction – are recommended. The use of high-efficacy particulate (HEPA) filters should be an effective means of decreasing the incidence of *Aspergillus* infection (see below). Certain foodstuffs, such as cereals, nuts and spices, e.g. ground black pepper, have been found to be contaminated with aspergilli and should not be offered to patients at risk of developing invasive pulmonary aspergillosis. However, the principles of environmental control of nosocomial aspergillosis are complex given that even HEPA units are not completely effective in preventing disease. Fungal exposure would be more precisely studied using a personal air sampler for the patient, but there is no fungal sampler currently available that can be used in this way, and there are also severe technical limitations on the duration of the sampling time of available fungal samplers.

The relationship between aspergillosis in predisposed patients and building work is also complex. Hospitals are buildings of continuous change and adaptation, so construction is an inevitable prospect which may extend throughout the year. Whether or not this activity is complicated by an outbreak of infection in the susceptible patients nearby, or is a risk related directly to the amount of disruption or some other factor, is unknown.

Currently, the environmental mycology of most outbreaks of nosocomial aspergillosis is poorly defined. However, the development of molecular biology techniques more directly applicable to *Aspergillus* spp. may help resolve some of these difficulties.

Aspergillus spp. have a major reservoir in organic debris, bird droppings, dust and building material. The principal approach to the prevention of aspergillosis is to minimise patients' exposure to *Aspergillus* conidia by filtering air or initiating some form of patient isolation. In some instances surface disinfection with copper-8-quinolinolate has been reported to be effective. Susceptible patients should not be treated in areas where there is construction or demolition activity, and if such activities are under way, measures should be instigated to seal these sites to prevent air exchange with the patients' environment.

Although outbreaks of invasive aspergillosis have been associated with construction within or around a hospital, the precise source of the fungus is occasionally difficult to trace with certainty. There have been few studies that have prospectively examined the aeromycology in and around a hospital during major building alterations and then compared these findings with samples from patients and the incidence of invasive aspergillosis.

In a seminal study the investigators took advantage of the opportunities that arose during widespread building operations around their hospital where several groups of patients seemed at risk of fungal infection: in wards for renal transplantation, bone marrow transplantation, oncology and intensive care (Goodley *et al.* 1994). Air samples were taken in these wards (by SAS Sampler, pbi International, Milan, Italy) and various outdoor sites around the hospital, at specific sites throughout the hospital, sequentially throughout the year as well as in particular areas during periods of construction activity. Nasal swabs were also taken from patients for comparison with the air sampling results. The most commonly isolated fungal species was *A. fumigatus*. Nasal swabs were positive in 12 of 188 samples—11 *A. fumigatus* and one *A. sydowi*. Most of the air samples cultured less than 10 cfu/m^3 throughout the year. A peak of higher counts occurred in March (190 cfu/m^3, confirmed at various sites) which could not be explained either by building work or by meteorology. Eight of the positive nasal swabs were obtained during March; three cases of invasive aspergillosis developed through the year and did not seem to be related to the spell of higher spore counts. One of the buildings was demolished, but there was no significant rise in spore counts and no change in the background pattern of fungal isolation in the wards or the corridors. Air sampling was repeated over the following year when a peak was recorded in June at 90 cfu/m^3, and very similar low levels throughout the rest of the year. The authors' interpretation of the results was that, because cases of invasive aspergillosis seemed to develop at low spore levels, then all highly susceptible patients should have protective isolation (HEPA ventilation and sterile management procedures). Routine nasal swab sampling was not proposed as an alternative to air sampling. Avoidance measures appear to be appropriate if minimal exposure is the only component necessary to induce invasive aspergillosis in transplant recipients.

Many of the environmental hazards contributing to invasive aspergillosis have been identified, including unfiltered air, defects in hospital ventilation systems, food items, and possibly hospital water supplies. Stringent environmental controls in transplant units have included high-efficiency air filtration, positive-pressure ventilation and frequent room-air changes. Although there have been several well-documented examples of aspergillosis outbreaks as a result of hospital demolition and reconstruction, it has not always been possible to demonstrate elevated spore counts in clinical areas during building work. Furthermore, the possibility of community-acquired aspergillosis must be considered. These risks can usually be effectively minimized. However, very few studies have linked environmental exposure to cases of invasive aspergillosis.

Thus, for optimal quality of care, preventative measures based on elimination of *Aspergillus* and other fungal spores from the environment of such patients is of paramount importance. In hospitals there are various strategies for preventing invasive aspergillosis (IA).

1. Protection of patients at very high risk of *Aspergillus* infection in rooms equipped with HEPA and laminar air flow (LAF) and implementation of specific preventive measures when renovation, construction or maintenance works are done in the hospital.
2. Regular environmental control of fungal contamination in isolation units and prospective surveillance of IA cases to detect any abnormal situation.
3. An understanding of the potential sources of *Aspergillus* conidia.

In addition to developing strategies to avoid exposure to fungal spores it is equally important to determine whether patients acquire their infection while in hospital or in their home environment. During the past ten years investigators have attempted to determine a link between the occurrence of IA in hospitalised patients and fungal contamination of the home/work environment, and to understand further the epidemiology of this infection. Two strategies have been explored:

1. Molecular methods have been used to determine where patients acquired IA, to answer the question: is the infection community- or hospital-acquired? All the studies reported so far have highlighted the limits of molecular biology to certify

the contamination sources. The molecular epidemiology of aspergillosis is complex. Given the ecology and biodiversity of *Aspergillus fumigatus* and the practical difficulties in obtaining representative environmental samples, hoping to identify the source of the fungus is more or less impossible. There are notable exceptions: faulty vacuum cleaners, pigeon excreta, etc.

2. Another approach has been the longitudinal surveillance of protected and non-protected areas in haematology units with follow-up of IA cases in an attempt to test the possibility that measuring air and sampling the hospital environment can be used to assess the risk of *Aspergillus* infection.

Many studies have demonstrated the efficacy of LAF plus HEPA filtration and HEPA filtration alone in preventing environmental *Aspergillus* contamination during hospital renovation (see, for example, Barnes & Rogers 1989; Kennedy *et al.* 1995). To show the usefulness of environmental surveillance to facilitate protection of patients at risk for invasive pulmonary aspergillosis Cornet *et al.* (1999) performed prospective sampling of air and surfaces for *Aspergillus* conidia during a 2-year period in a haematology department adjacent to building renovation at a university hospital. A total of 1047 air samples and 1178 surface samples were collected from January 1996 to December 1997. Significantly more air samples were positive for *Aspergillus* species during the period of building renovation than during the periods before and after renovation in a unit without a protected air supply adjacent to the building work area (51.5% versus 31.7%; odds ratio (OR), 2.3; 95% confidence interval (C195%), 1.4–3.7; $p < 0.001$). A major increase in the frequency of positive air samples was also found in another adjacent unit that was protected with HEPA filtration alone (from 1.8% to 47.5%; OR, 48.9; C195, 12–229; $p < 10^{-7}$). In addition, in this unit, the mean count of *Aspergillus* conidia in positive air samples increased significantly during construction (4–24.7 cfu/m^3; $p = 0.04$) and the proportion of positive surface samples showed a significant increase during renovation (from 0.4% to 9.7%; OR, 28.3; C195%, 3.4–623; $p = 10^{-4}$). However, none of 142 air samples collected during renovation in the area protected with LAF plus HEPA filtration showed *Aspergillus* conidia. In a unit distant from the building renovation site, the results of air and surface samples were not affected by renovation. The authors concluded that their study showed a strong association between building renovation and an increase in environmental *Aspergillus* contamination and that the results confirmed the high efficacy of LAF plus HEPA filtration and a high air-change rate. Although filtration with HEPA was effective during normal conditions, it alone was unable to prevent the rise of *Aspergillus* contamination related to building renovation. The study emphasized the necessity for an environmental survey of airborne contamination related to construction to facilitate prevention of nosocomial aspergillosis outbreaks and that a standardized protocol for aerobiological surveillance is needed.

Oren *et al.* (2001) reported that between September and December 1993, during extensive hospital construction and indoor renovation, a nosocomial outbreak of invasive pulmonary aspergillosis occurred in acute leukaemia patients treated in a regular ward that had only natural ventilation. The observed infection rate was 50%. Chemoprophylaxis with intravenous continuous low-dose amphotericin B was then instituted as a preventive measure. During the next 18 months, invasive pulmonary aspergillosis developed in 43% of acute leukaemia patients. After that period a new haematology ward was opened with an air filtration system through HEPA filters, and a bone marrow transplantation programme was started on the haematology service. During the next three years, none of the acute leukaemia or bone marrow transplantation patients who were hospitalized exclusively in the haematology ward developed invasive pulmonary aspergillosis, although 29% of acute leukaemia patients who were housed in a regular ward, because of shortage of space in the new facility, still contracted invasive pulmonary aspergillosis. Overall, 31 patients were diagnosed with invasive pulmonary aspergillosis during almost five years: 74% of patients recovered from invasive pulmonary aspergillosis, and 42% are long-term survivors; 26% of patients died of resistant leukaemia with aspergillosis, but no-one died of invasive pulmonary aspergillosis alone. This study confirmed previous findings that by keeping patients in facilities with HEPA-filtered air eliminates invasive pulmonary aspergillosis completely.

Other recent studies confirm these conclusions. Alberti *et al.* (2001) prospectively examined the relationship between environmental contamination by *Aspergillus* and other fungal species and the incidence of invasive nosocomial aspergillosis (INA) in a bone marrow transplantation unit and two haematology wards. During a four-year period, levels of air and surface fungal contamination were determined bi-monthly in patients' rooms (some equipped with HEPA filters and LAF systems), and various common sites in each ward (corridors, nursing stations, etc.). Results were compared with the incidence of INA. A total of 3100 air and 9800 surface samples were collected, and 79 cases of IA were diagnosed, of which 64 were probably or possibly INA. Patterns of fungal contamination were comparable in the three wards, with a gradient ranging from high levels in common sites to a virtual absence in rooms equipped with HEPA filters and LAF systems. Using a regression model, a significant relationship was found between the incidence of INA and the degree of fungal contamination of air and surfaces in conventional patient rooms (not equipped with HEPA) and common sites. This study shows that in a non-epidemic setting, there is a significant relationship between environmental fungal contamination in haematology wards and the incidence of INA. The authors conclude that their findings emphasise the importance of environmental surveillance and strict application of preventive measures.

In a neonatal intensive care unit Mahieu *et al.* (2000) determined the relationship between air contamination by *Aspergillus* spp., in three renovation areas of a neonatal intensive care unit (NICU) and colonisation and infection rates in a high-care area (HC) equipped with HEPA filtration and a high-pressure system. Data on the type and site of renovation works, outdoor meteorological conditions, patient crowding and nasopharyngeal colonization rate were collected. Factors not associated with *Aspergillus* spp. concentration were outdoor temperature, air pressure, wind speed, humidity, rainfall, patient density in the NICU, and renovation works in the administrative area and in the isolation rooms. Multivariate analysis revealed that renovation works and air concentration of *Aspergillus* spp. spores in the medium-care area (MC) resulted in a significant increase of the concentration in the HC of the NICU. The use of a mobile HEPA air filtration system caused a significant decrease in the *Aspergillus* spp. concentration. There was no relationship between *Aspergillus* spp. air concentration and nasopharyngeal colonization in the neonates. Invasive aspergillosis did not occur during the renovation. This study highlights the importance of optimal physical barriers and air filtration to decrease airborne fungal spores in high-risk units during renovation works. However, the value of patient surveillance and environmental air sampling is questionable because no relationship was found between air contamination and colonization in patients.

Sources of infection

Numerous studies have attempted to define specific sources of *Aspergillus* conidia. Several illustrative investigations are presented here.

The spectrum and concentration of fungal species in hospital environments varies considerably from institution to institution and within different locations in individual hospitals. Rainer *et al.* (2001) monitored the biodiversity and concentration of airborne fungi over 6 months in a special-care unit. Air sampling was done in a corridor that was also accessible to visitors and in an adjacent bone-marrow transplantation (BMT) unit using an air sampler and two isolation media. Altogether, 98 fungal species were identified, among them *A. fumigatus* and *A. terreus* as well as 48 other species reported as potential pathogens. The average contamination values of the corridor air ranged from 124 to 485 cfu/m^3. Neither the degree of fungal air contamination nor the species composition inside the special care unit differed from those found in the corridor. Data obtained with a light-activated sensor showed a possible influence of human activities on diurnal changes of fungal propagule concentration.

In a paediatric oncology ward all cases of aspergillosis were identified from the hospital records and categorised as definite or probable according to the extent of supportive clinical and laboratory findings (Anderson *et al.* 1996). All relevant aspects of building ventilation, air filtration and aerosol generation considered relevant were examined and air samples for fungi were taken in triplicate at 25 sites. Six cases of aspergillosis were identified over one year out of the 148 patients who attended the unit—the only part of the hospital where cases were found. Examination of the building services and function suggested that the cause or source was isolated to this paediatric oncology/haematology ward and may have been attributed to a defective disposal conduit door as well as the dispersal of a contaminated aerosol from the ward vacuum cleaner which had the highest measured concentrations of *Aspergillus fumigatus* in or around the building (65 cfu/m^3 compared with 0–6 cfu/m^3 elsewhere). No further cases were identified in the two years after these hygiene arrangements were changed. The investigation of this outbreak of nosocomial aspergillosis identified several possible sources of contaminated aerosols which could have been implicated as the cause. Their modification was followed by a reduction in the incidence of further cases.

Water has also been implicated as a source of *Aspergillus*. To determine whether water or water-related surfaces are a reservoir for opportunistic filamentous fungi, water sampling in the paediatric BMT unit of the National Hospital University of Oslo, Norway, Warris *et al.* (2001) analysed over a six-month period 168 water samples and 20 samples from water-related surfaces. The water samples were taken from the taps and showers in the BMT unit and from the main pipe supplying the paediatric department with water. In addition, 20 water samples were taken at the intake reservoir supplying the city of Oslo with drinking water. Filamentous fungi were recovered from 94% of all the water samples taken inside the hospital with a mean cfu count of 2.7/500 mL of water. *A. fumigatus* was recovered from 49% and 5.6% of water samples from the taps and showers, respectively (mean 1.9 and 1.0 cfu per 500 mL). More than one third (38.8%) of water samples from the main pipe revealed *A. fumigatus* (mean 2.1 cfu per 500 mL). All water samples taken at the intake reservoir were culture positive for filamentous fungi; 85% of the water samples showed *A. fumigatus* (mean 3.1 cfu per 500 mL). Twenty-five percent of water-related surfaces yielded filamentous fungi, but *A. fumigatus* was recovered from only two samples. The study showed that filamentous fungi are present in the hospital water and to a lesser extent on water-related surfaces. The recovery of filamentous fungi in water samples taken at the intake reservoir suggests that the source of contamination is located outside the hospital.

A further study from Greece emphasises that hospital water supplies could be a potential source of *Aspergillus* conidia (Arvanitidou *et al.* 1999). The prevalence of fungi was investigated in 126 potable water samples (84 hospital and 42 community samples), in parallel with the standard pollution indicator microorganisms. Filamentous fungi were isolated from 104 of 126 (82.5%) samples and yeasts from 14 (11.1%), whereas their mean counts were 36.6 and 4.4, respectively. Fungi were isolated from 95.2% of community and 76.2% of hospital water samples, with the difference being statistically significant ($p < 0.05$), whereas yeasts were isolated from 9.5 and 11.9%, respectively. Prevailing genera were *Penicillium* spp., isolated from 64, *Aspergillus* spp. from 53, and *Candida* from 9, of the examined samples. Colony-forming units of yeasts were significantly correlated with those of total and faecal coliforms, whereas the counts of filamentous fungi were significantly correlated with total heterotrophic bacteria counts. These results suggest that tap water is a potential transmission route for fungi both in hospitals and the community in the examined region and may pose a health hazard mainly for the immunocompromised host.

Arvanitidou *et al.* (2000) have also reported their analysis of treated water and the dialysate from all 85 haemodialysis units in Greece, to estimate the occurrence of fungi. Filamentous fungi and yeasts were isolated from 69 (81.2%) and from 3 (3.5%) feed-water samples, from 74 (87.1%) and 7 (8.2%) treated water samples and from 66 (77.7%) and 11 (12.9%) dialysate samples respectively. *Aspergillus* spp. and *Penicillium* spp. were the most frequent moulds. Counts of filamentous fungi in all 255 samples were significantly correlated with the counts of total heterotrophic bacteria and enterococci, whereas the counts of yeasts were correlated with faecal coliforms, total heterotrophic bacteria, as well as enterococci, *Pseudomonas* spp. and total coliforms, whereas no correlation was detected with the age of either haemodialysis units, the age of water treatment system, the number of artificial kidney machines or the components of the water purification system. High recovery of fungi from haemodialysis aqueous environments implies a potential risk for haemodialysis patients and indicates the need for continuous maintenance and monitoring.

Further studies from the USA illustrate the potential of hospital water supplies as a major source of nosocomial aspergillosis (Anaissie & Costa 2001; Anaissie *et al.* 2002).

Aspergillus species are frequently present on food and thus may be an indirect source of airway or digestive tract colonisation. Many different foods have long been recognised as potential sources of *Aspergillus* conidia. A recent study showed that conidia were cultured from 100% of pepper and tea samples, 12–66% of fruits, 27% of herbal teas, and 20% of freeze-dried soup samples (Bouakline *et al.* 2000).

Risk assessment

To avoid patients being exposed to nosocomial fungal pathogens it is of paramount importance to conduct a risk assessment of the hospital facility where high-risk patients are being managed. The process of risk assessment includes the steps of hazard identification, exposure assessment, and dose response assessment, drawn together as a hazard analysis or risk characterisation. Risk management strategies can then be implemented after this process. There is, however, very little published work on the application of formal risk assessment models in nosocomial fungal infection.

Many of the agents of nosocomial infection are normal inhabitants of the environment, hence nosocomial infection can be thought of broadly as an environmental health problem and many of the risk assessment techniques used to investigate the risks associated with environmental contaminants such as toxic chemicals may be applied to microbiological hazards. This has already been successfully accomplished in the assessment of microbiological hazards in food and drinking water. There are, however, several major difficulties in the application of formal risk assessment methods to the quantification of microbiological risk, as summarised in a recent report by the UK Advisory Committee on Dangerous Pathogens (ACDP 1996). These difficulties will be highlighted at appropriate points during the following discussion (modified from Wilkinson 1998).

Microbial risk assessment

This is defined by the UK Advisory Committee on Dangerous Pathogens as a 'formal structured procedure for identifying and characterising microbiological hazard and determining the risk associated with it.' Risk analysis is a structured approach to the reduction of risk (see Introduction). This process involves the calculation of both the probability and impact of disease. The management of risk then involves the examination of ways in which either the probability of disease or its severity can be reduced. An important part of the whole process is the communication of the level of risk to the community at large and to those sections of the population considered to be most 'at risk' of the adverse health outcome. Surveillance and monitoring of outcomes is also important to assess the effectiveness of risk management strategies. Some of the benefits of this approach are to assist policy makers in the design of risk management (infection control) practices, and to highlight current inadequacies in the scientific basis of microbial risk assessment.

Hazard identification

This involves a qualitative assessment of whether a threat to patients exists and formulation of exposure pathways based on an evaluation of available epidemiological and clinical evidence. Several lines of evidence suggest that inhalation of airborne fungal spores causes aspergillosis in susceptible individuals. One report describes at least 25 nosocomial outbreaks of aspergillosis (Walsh & Dixon 1989). In all instances where an aetiology could be discerned, there was either a breakdown in the hospital ventilation system, building construction or some other disruption that rendered settled spores airborne, or the presence of an in-hospital source of airborne *Aspergillus* spores. Anderson *et al.* (1996) described a series of six cases of invasive aspergillosis in paediatric haematology/oncology patients where the focus of spread of fungal spores was thought to be the ward vacuum cleaner.

Exposure assessment

This involves a measurement or prediction of the amount and duration of exposure to the hazard, in this case the number of viable *Aspergillus* spp. spores inhaled. Consideration needs to be given to the range of host susceptibilities as well as the potential pathogenicity of the microbe. There is little information on differences in pathogenicity between different strains of *Aspergillus* spp. in the hospital setting. Most cases of nosocomially acquired *Aspergillus* infection occur in the severely immunocompromised. These types of patient are generally seen in tertiary-care hospitals and may form up to 10% of the inpatient population, depending on the specialties of the hospital.

Respiratory aspergillosis results from endobronchial germination of inhaled spores (conidia) and subsequent proliferation of hyphae. The size of *A. fumigatus* conidia (approximately 2–3.5 μm) facilitates their deposition throughout the tracheobronchial tree whereas the smaller particles may be deposited in the alveoli. About half of particles in the range 2–5 μm impact in the upper respiratory tract (Rhame 1991). Therefore it should be possible to calculate the periodic exposure to *Aspergillus* in the hospital environment using a calculation of the number of viable spores in ambient air multiplied by the average respiratory volume. The minute respiratory volume is considered to be about 6 L/min in healthy young men (Schottelius & Schottelius 1978), and if this is taken as an average figure for the population at risk, this equates to the inhalation of approximately 480 L, or 0.48 m^3, of air per hour. The number of *Aspergillus* spores present in normal outside air varies considerably with geographical location and season. Therefore, to make a meaningful quantitative estimation of exposure it would be necessary to have access to local data on *Aspergillus* spore counts. As an illustration, we know from several studies that the average viable spore count in normal ward air ranges from 1 to 40 cfu/m^3 of air. Taking a median level of 20 cfu/m^3 would indicate an average hourly exposure of $20 \times 0.48 = 9.6$ viable spores. However, only a proportion of these spores are likely to impact on the lower airway, possibly about 50% (see above). Therefore, there is an average hourly exposure of approximately 5 viable *Aspergillus* spp. spores.

In practice such quantitative estimates are very difficult to make because many factors intervene, such as the reliability of sampling air for fungal propagules (see below), the range of values for the minute respiratory volume for different individuals, and the degree of susceptibility of individuals to infection. Also, molecular typing techniques that enable definitive linking of cases of aspergillosis to environmental isolates have only recently become available (Leenders *et al.* 1996). In addition, *Aspergillus* spp. spores are often only periodically shed into the air, usually after some environmental disturbance. This makes estimates of average spore counts problematical and highly uncertain.

Dose–response relationship

The next important step in attempting to define exposure and risk is to examine the dose–response relationship. There are very few animal studies that are applicable to the assessment of dose–response with *Aspergillus* spp. However, it may be concluded (tentatively) from the above that a normal healthy person's immune system is able to cope with an hourly challenge of around 5 viable spores. However, when the immune system is impaired, this number presents a significant risk of disease.

Probably the best source of information on dose–response for *Aspergillus* spp. pneumonia is the study by Arnow *et al.* (1991). Their study involved the regular monthly collection of air samples and active case surveillance over 6 years. They reported an incidence of 0.3% which rose to 1.2% during the epidemic period.

Aspergillus spp. spore counts were found to be ≤0.2 cfu/m^3 of air initially, rising to 1.1–2.2 cfu/m^3 during the epidemic period. Rhame *et al.* (1984) reported a risk of 5.4% when the mean concentration of *A. fumigatus* in patients' rooms was 0.9 cfu/m^3, and Sherertz *et al.* (1987) reported no cases of aspergillosis in 39 patients when levels of *Aspergillus* spp. spores were reduced to 0.009 cfu/m^3. Thus a spore level of <0.1 cfu/m^3 is likely to be required to reduce the risk to below 0.1% in susceptible patients. Using the same calculation as above, 0.1 cfu/m^3 represents an hourly challenge of only 0.048 spores. Therefore, a susceptible patient would need many hours of exposure to receive a dose of only one *Aspergillus* spore. However, as previously mentioned, fungal spores are often shed into the air in bursts. This indicates there is no 'safe' level for these patients and every effort should be taken to remove *Aspergillus* spp. spores from the air.

These figures should be interpreted with caution. The detection of *Aspergillus* spores in the air supply is accomplished by air sampling. There are many designs of air sampling machines, which vary considerably in their performance characteristics (Morris *et al.* 2000). Some types sample air directly onto agar plates either through a sieve or a small slit; others make use of centrifugal force to deposit particles onto an agar strip or into liquid broth, and yet another type draws air through a micropore filter (usually 0.45 μm pore size) and the filter is placed onto the surface of an agar plate for incubation. Each method has its strengths and weaknesses and different situations may require different sampling methods. There is little published data on the range of particle sizes sampled and the relative efficiencies of the various methods. The choice of air sampling method, particularly the volume and speed of air sampling, is critical for the evaluation of published data on airborne microbial levels.

In addition, although air sampling is a method for counting the number of viable spores, it does not give a measure of the pathogenicity of the isolates. Such assessment requires the use of molecular techniques, which have not been applied systematically to this problem as yet. Thus, any reliable quantitative assessment of infective dose is at present difficult to obtain. More research is needed in this area.

Risk characterisation

This is the process of drawing together the information gained by hazard analysis and exposure assessment, with any information available on the dose–response relationship, to present an overall picture of the hazard. This can then form the basis for making decisions about the management of the hazard and minimisation of the risk to public health.

In invasive aspergillosis in immunocompromised patients, the hazard has been identified as the inhalation of viable spores of *Aspergillus* spp. (mostly *A. fumigatus* and *A. flavus*), coupled with a high degree of immunosuppression. The patients most at risk are those with haematological malignancies, particularly those undergoing bone marrow transplantation, and other cancer patients on immunosuppressive treatment. There are currently insufficient data to perform a meaningful quantitative risk assessment for this disease, but extrapolation from disease outbreak reports among susceptible patients indicates that the infective dose may be very low, and inhalation of a single spore may give rise to a significant risk of infection.

One of the most difficult aspects of this assessment is the ability to accurately measure very low infective spore concentrations in air. It is necessary to measure at least 10 m^3 of air for each sample, but there are very few machines that are designed to draw such large samples. Although most of the published studies have concentrated on the air supply as the potential source of spores, it may well be that spores are more likely to be introduced into the patient's environment by human activity. An experimental study by Buttner & Stetzenbach (1993) has shown significantly higher airborne spore concentrations after human activity in a controlled experimental environment. They also demonstrated that the level of repeatability was low overall for aerobiological samplers, suggesting that a single air sample at a single location may have limited value.

Risk management

Microbiological risk assessment methods assist in the determination of guidelines to assist infection control practitioners in developing appropriate risk management strategies, and in providing the scientific basis for communicating the rationale behind such measures. There are currently no published numerical guidelines for *Aspergillus* spore counts in air, although local experience suggests that there should be fewer than 0.1 cfu/m^3 in HEPA-filtered air. This, however, leaves the problem of inaccuracy of sampling at such very low levels, as previously mentioned. The most recent guidelines on the prevention of nosocomial pneumonia published by the Centers for Disease Control and Prevention (1997) outlines measures aimed at the reduction of exposure levels to *Aspergillus* spp. spores by the installation of HEPA filters in high-risk patients' rooms, coupled with positive air pressure and high rates of room-air changes. They give no recommendation for performing routine, periodic cultures of air samples, ventilation ducts and filters in rooms occupied by high-risk patients, and declare this an 'unresolved issue'.

HEPA filters are 99.97% efficient in filtering particles ≥0.3 μm in diameter. Use of these filters, properly installed and maintained, should reduce the theoretical exposure rate of 5 spores per hour to 0.0015 spores per hour. Because the volume of air inspired in one hour is approximately 0.48 m^3, this represents a concentration of approximately 0.003 spores per cubic metre of air. The study by Sherertz *et al.* (1987) indicated that, at average spore counts of 0.009 per cubic metre, no cases of invasive aspergillosis were found among their 39 high-risk patients.

In addition to air filtration, consideration should be given to other potential sources of *Aspergillus* within the hospital, because these may become foci for fungal colonisation and the release of bursts of spores into the air. These may then be carried into the rooms of high-risk patients by persons entering the room. Patients should also be protected by well-fitting masks when being transported to other areas of the hospital to undergo diagnostic and other procedures.

Communication

The process of risk management involves communication with building and air-conditioning engineers to ensure that the special needs of high-risk patients are understood, and the need for regular maintenance and testing of the integrity of the filters is appreciated. There should be put in place a regular review of maintenance practices by the Infection Control Committee. Although regular monitoring of the air supply is probably not warranted, routine surveillance of infections in these groups of patients is very important to detect the possible occurrence of an outbreak. In such a case, environmental monitoring is required to establish whether there has been a breakdown in the maintenance system.

Hospital policies should also be formulated to minimise the risk of exposure to higher than normal levels of spores during construction and renovation activities. This requires the input of the hospital engineers, the nursing and medical directors of the Haematology and Cancer units, the hospital administrator and the Infection Control Committee.

Nursing and medical staff should be educated in the special risks faced by the immunocompromised patient from the normal environment. This is usually the function of the Infection Control Practitioner or Hospital Epidemiologist. In addition, patients should be made aware of the potential risks they face from normal environmental organisms when undergoing immunosuppressive treatments. This is normally the responsibility of the treating physician.

In conclusion, at this time, there is insufficient experimental and epidemiological data on nosocomial aspergillosis to conduct a fully quantitative microbial risk assessment, and therefore to fully assess the impact of this disease on hospitalised patients. However, the strategies that are currently recommended focus on the minimisation of risk by the removal of potential sources of *Aspergillus* spores from the high-risk patient's environment.

To summarise, there are several factors that prevent the universal implementation of this strategy.

1. The lack of standardized methods to investigate fungal biocontamination.
2. The absence of normal values and threshold levels of *Aspergillus* and other filamentous fungi contamination adjusted to the degree of immunosuppression in patients.
3. Difficulties in assessing the nosocomial character of IA because little is known about the relationship between the time of fungal exposure and occurrence of disease.

A proposed surveillance model for monitoring the aerobiology of hospital environments

The application of a longitudinal sampling programme for fungal contamination of hospital environments has previously been reported (Richardson *et al.* 2000). The use of this model is illustrated further by a 7-week surveillance programme in the liver and kidney transplant units of Helsinki University Central Hospital (unpublished observations). Fifteen different locations in open wards and central areas in each unit were monitored weekly for pathogenic fungi by: (1) mycological and immunological analysis of dust that had been collected continuously during the previous 7 days; (2) by contact plate sampling of surfaces; (3) by sampling 1000 L of air using an SAS Super-100 impactor; and (4) by mycological and immunological analysis of hot and cold water supplies. Immunological analysis of dust extracts and water samples was done by using the Platelia *Aspergillus* enzyme-linked immunosorbent assay (ELISA) for galactomannan antigen. During the 7-week programme, significant numbers of *Aspergillus fumigatus* were found in dust from bedrooms, corridors and toilet facilities although there was considerable variation in colony forming units from week-to-week. In contrast, very few *A. fumigatus* conidia were detected in air or water samples. Low levels of galactomannan antigen were detected in dust but not in water. The results of this study highlight the utility of dust collection and analysis in monitoring hospital environments for pathogenic fungi. There were no conclusive cases of invasive aspergillosis during or immediately after this study was done. It is proposed that this model could be become an integral part of hospital infection control.

References

ACDP (1996). *Microbiological risk assessment: an interim report.* London, Advisory Committee on Dangerous Pathogens.

Alberti C, Bouakline A *et al.* (2001). Relationship between environmental fungal contamination and the incidence of invasive aspergillosis in haematology patients. *Journal of Hospital Infection* **48**, 198–206.

Anaissie EJ, Costa SF (2001). Nosocomila aspergillosis is waterborne. *Clinical Infectious Diseases* **33**, 1546–1548.

Anaissie EJ, Stratton SL, Dignani MC *et al.* (2002). Cleaning patient shower facilities: a novel approach to reducing patient exposure to aerosolized *Aspergillus* species and other opportunistic molds. *Clinical Infectious Diseases* **35**, e86–e88.

Anderson K, Morris G *et al.* (1996). Aspergillosis in immunocompromised paediatric patients: associations with building hygiene, design, and indoor air. *Thorax* **51**, 256–261.

Arnow PM, Sadigh M *et al.* (1991). Endemic and epidemic aspergillosis associated with in-hospital replication of *Aspergillus* organisms. *Journal of Infectious Diseases* **164**, 998–1002.

Arvanitidou M, Spaia S *et al.* (2000). High level of recovery of fungi from water and dialysate in haemodialysis units. *Journal of Hospital Infection* **45**, 225–230.

Arvanitidou M, Kanellou K *et al.* (1999). The occurrence of fungi in hospital and community potable waters. *Letters in Applied Microbiology* **29**, 81–84.

Barnes RA, Rogers TR (1989). Control of an outbreak of nosocomial aspergillosis by laminar air-flow isolation. *Journal of Hospital Infection* **14**, 89–94.

Bouakline A, Lacroix C *et al.* (2000). Fungal contamination of food in haematology units. *Journal of Clinical Microbiology* **38**, 4272–4273.

Buttner MP & Stetzenbach LD (1993). Monitoring airborne fungal spores in an experimental indoor environment to evaluate sampling methods and the effects of human activity on air sampling. *Applied and Environmental Microbiology* **59**, 219–226.

Centers for Disease Control and Prevention (1997). Guidelines for prevention of nosocomial pneumonia. *Morbidity and Mortality Weekly Report* **46** (No. RR-1), 58–62.

Cornet M, Levy V *et al.* (1999). Efficacy of prevention by high-efficiency particulate air filtration or laminar airflow against *Aspergillus* airborne contamination during hospital renovation. *Journal of Hospital Infection* **20**, 508–513.

Ellis M, Richardson MD, de Pauw B (2000). Epidemiology of systemic fungal infection. *Hospital Medicine* **61**, 605–609.

Goodley JM, Clayton YM, Hay RJ (1994). Environmental sampling for aspergilli during building construction on a hospital site. *Journal of Hospital Infection* **26**, 27–35.

Kennedy HF, Michie JR, Richardson MD (1995). Air sampling for *Aspergillus* spp. during building activity in a paediatric hospital ward. *Journal of Hospital Infection* **32**, 259–263.

Leenders A, van Belkum A *et al.* (1996). Molecular epidemiology of apparent outbreak of invasive aspergillosis in a haematology ward. *Journal of Clinical Microbiology* **34,** 345–351.

Manuel RJ, Kibbler CC (1998). The epidemiology and prevention of invasive aspergillosis. *Journal of Hospital Infection* **39**, 95–109.

Mahieu LM, De Dooy JJ *et al.* (2000). A prospective study on factors influencing *Aspergillus* spore load in the air during renovation works in a neonatal intensive care unit. *Journal of Hospital Infection* **45**, 191–197.

Morris G, Kokki MH, Anderson K, Richardson MD (2000). Sampling of *Aspergillus* spores in air. *Journal of Hospital Infection* **44**, 81–92.

Oren I, Haddard N *et al.* (2001). Invasive pulmonary aspergillosis in neutropenic patients during hospital construction: before and after chemoprophylaxis and institution of HEPA filters. *American Journal of Hematology* **66**, 257–262.

Rainer J, Peintner U, Poder R (2001). Biodiversity and concentration of airborne fungi in a hospital environment. *Mycopathologia* **149**, 87–97.

Rhame FS (1991). Prevention of nosocomial aspergillosis. *Journal of Hospital Infection* **18** (Suppl A), 466–472.

Rhame FS, Streifel AJ *et al.* (1984). Extrinsic risk factors for pneumonia in the patient at high risk of infection. *American Journal of Medicine* **76** (Suppl. 5A), 45–52.

Richardson MD, Rennie S *et al.* (2000). Fungal surveillance of an open haematology ward. *Journal of Hospital Infection* **44**, 1–5.

Richardson MD, Kokki MH (1998). Prevention and diagnosis of systemic fungal infections in immunocompromised patients. *Blood Reviews* **12**, 241–254.

Richardson MD, Kokki MH (1999). New perspectives in the diagnosis of systemic fungal infections. *Annals of Medicine* **31**, 327–335.

Richardson MD, Ellis M (2000). Clinical and laboratory diagnosis of systemic fungal infection. *Hospital Medicine* **61**, 610–614.

Richardson MD, Kokki MH (2002). Aspergillus. In: *Clinical Mycology* (eds E Anaissie, MR McGinnis, MA Pfaller). Churchill Livingstone, New York.

Schottelius BA, Schottelius DD (1978). Gas exchange – respiration. In *Textbook of Physiology* pp. 346–349. C.V. Mosby, Saint Louis.

Sherertz RJ, Belani A *et al.* (1987). Impact of air filtration on nosocomial *Aspergillus* infections: unique risk of bone marrow trnsplant recipients. *American Journal of Medicine* **83**, 709–718.

Walsh TJ, Dixon DM (1989). Nosocomial aspergillosis: environmental microbiology, hospital epidemiology, diagnosis and treatment. *European Journal of Epidemiology* **5**, 131–142.

Warnock DW, Hajjeh RA, Lasker BA (2001). Epidemiology and prevention of invasive aspergillosis. *Current Infectious Disease Reports* **3**, 507–516.

Warris A, Gaustad P *et al.* (2001). Recovery of filamentous fungi from water in a paediatric bone marrow transplantation unit. *Journal of Hospital Infection* **47**, 143–148.

Wilkinson I (1998). The application of a quantitative risk assessment paradigm to the acquisition of nosocomial infection caused by *Aspergillus* species. Master of Public Health thesis.

Chapter 3

Evaluating risk factors for invasive candidiasis in neutropenic patients in terms of the role of the gut

NMA Blijlevens and JP Donnelly

Introduction

Invasive candidiasis is a major cause of infectious complications related to cytotoxic treatment and conditioning regimens used for haematopoietic stem cell transplantation (HSCT). Although neutropenia is known to be an important risk factor, the damage to the epithelium of the intestinal tract, so-called mucosal barrier injury (MBI), has been largely ignored. When the gut is colonised by *Candida* species and damaged by cytotoxic therapy, this creates a portal of entry for the yeast. There is a relationship between MBI and colonisation on the one hand, and the onset of invasive candidiasis on the other. Methods for determining gut MBI made manifest by impairment of gut integrity and altered gut permeability are discussed and might prove useful for identifying patients at high risk for invasive disease. Such patients will be those treated for acute leukaemia with a regimen containing anthracyclines or high-dose cytarabine, as well as those receiving a haematopoietic stem cell (HSC) transplant after total body irradiation (TBI). Such high-risk patients are the ones who are most likely to benefit from antifungal prophylaxis, and who would normally not require any additional measures for prevention.

Candida colonisation of the gut

It has been shown that colonisation with *Candida* species invariably precedes infection (Martino *et al.* 1989). Although there are no internationally accepted criteria for defining *Candida* colonisation, it is usually accepted that isolation of the same yeast from two consecutive specimens from the same site at different times, e.g. at 3–4 day intervals, or from two different sites at the same time represents colonisation. The number of yeasts in each millilitre of saliva or gram of faeces is also recognised as a risk factor for invasive disease with higher counts in either being associated with more frequent invasive disease (Guiot *et al.* 1996). Surveillance cultures are especially useful in the absence of *Candida* colonisation because they can be used as a negative predictor of invasive disease (Laverdiere *et al.* 2000; Sandford *et al.* 1980). The negative predictive value is even higher when the *a priori* change of prevalence of *Candida albicans* colonisation is high as it is among patients treated with intensive cytotoxic drugs or those prepared for an HSCT. By contrast, apparent colonisation with *Candida tropicalis* is highly predictive of disease (Sandford *et al.* 1980), which remains important as this species is responsible for more than 50% of breakthrough candidaemia in cancer patients (Viscoli *et al.* 1999). The use of antifungal prophylaxis like with fluconazole was significantly associated with the occurrence of non-*albicans* candidaemia, which accounted for 40% of episodes, although colonisation with non-*albicans Candida* species was also increased among patients treated with intensive cytotoxic chemotherapy for acute leukaemia and among recipients of an autologous HSCT, whether or not they had received the drug (Laverdiere *et al.* 2000). A higher rate of bacteraemia has also been observed among febrile neutropenic patients receiving antifungal prophylaxis (Viscoli *et al.* 2001) and the occurrence of invasive candidiasis appears related to both the onset of bacteraemia and the degree of *Candida* colonisation (Guiot *et al.* 1994).

However, the association between invasive candidiasis and bacteraemia may be indirect and the result of the selective pressure exerted as a result of the use of certain broad-spectrum β-lactam antibiotics with anaerobic activity such as piperacillin or imipenem because these drugs tend to impair the ecology of the lower gastrointestinal tract leading to an increase in yeast colonisation of the gastrointestinal tract (Samonis *et al.* 1993). It is also tempting to speculate that both infectious complications are the result of passage of the microorganism through the damaged gut mucosal barrier in these patients.

Cytotoxic-therapy-induced gut mucosal-barrier injury and invasive candidiasis

In mice, adherence of *C. albicans* to the gastrointestinal mucosa and systemic dissemination is increased after TBI and chemotherapy (Sandovsky-Losica & Segal *et al.* 1989, 1990, 1992). The inclusion of TBI in the myeloablative regimen for HSCT recipients also leads to more bacteraemia and invasive candidiasis (Verfaillie *et al.* 1991; Goodrich *et al.* 1991; Callum *et al.* 1991). Furthermore, patients undergoing induction chemotherapy for acute myeloid leukaemia with a regimen of either cytarabine plus an anthracycline or high-dose cytarabine are at greater risk of developing invasive candidiasis (Rotstein *et al.* 1999). The absorption of D-xylose significantly declines in weeks 2 and 3 after starting treatment with these regimens. The onset of bacteraemia, candidaemia or hepatosplenic candidiasis also corresponds with poor absorption of D-xylose (Bow *et al.* 1997, 1998), suggesting a clear role for gut MBI. Neutropenic enterocolitis, which is the most severe manifestation of gut MBI, is also strongly correlated with the development of candidaemia, affecting patients who also have significantly lower D-xylose absorption (Bow *et al.* 1997). Hence, the neutropenia and damage to the gut mucosal barrier induced by cytotoxic chemotherapy, with shifts in the adherent microflora after exposure to antibacterial prophylaxis or therapy, likely facilitates the development of neutropenic enterocolitis (Vlasveld *et al.* 1991; Micozzi *et al.* 1996; Seipelt *et al.* 1998).

Measuring gut mucosal barrier injury after intensive cytotoxic therapy

The nature of the myeloablative regimen has been shown to be the most significant determinant of the severity and progression of oral mucositis (Wardley *et al.* 2000). Oral mucositis is a complex pathobiological process representing far more than simply a toxicological side-effect. It consists of at least four successive phases known as: (1) an inflammatory phase; (2) an epithelial phase; (3) an ulcerative-bacteriological phase; and (4) a healing phase (Sonis 1998; Blijlevens *et al.* 2000). By analogy, the same may be true of the gut but, in contrast to the mouth, the symptoms and physical signs of gut damage are not specific enough and are often masked by the administration of morphine to relieve pain. There is also no appropriate scoring system that accurately describes the course and severity of intestinal mucosal damage. Non-invasive methods for assessing gastro-intestinal permeability *in vivo* are an accepted surrogate for gut disease or gut damage (Bjarnason *et al.* 1995) and may prove useful for determining intestinal MBI because the principal features are alterations in permeability and the loss of epithelial surface, e.g. integrity. Permeability can be measured by detecting the presence of test substances in blood or urine. The disaccharide (lactulose), monosaccharides (L-rhamnose, mannitol, 3-ortho-methylglucose (3-OMG)), various polymers of polyethylene glycol or ^{51}Cr-labelled ethylenediaminetetraacetic acid (^{51}Cr-EDTA) have proved useful for investigating a variety of different intestinal diseases (Bjarnason *et al.* 1995). However, the use of different sugar probes seems the most practical as they are safe and well tolerated and equally affected by bowel transit time, gastric emptying and renal function allowing the urinary excretion ratio to function as an index of intestinal permeability. Moreover, irrespective of the probe that is used, disturbed permeability reaches a maximum 10–14 days after starting cytotoxic chemotherapy followed by recovery during the consecutive 3–4 weeks (Johansson & Ekman 1997; Selby *et al.* 1984; Daenen *et al.* 1991; Fegan *et al.* 1990; Keefe *et al.* 1997; Parrilli *et al.* 1989). By employing lactulose to indicate paracellular transport, 3-OMG to measure ATP-dependent transcellular transport, D-xylose to detect carrier-mediated transcellular transport, and L-rhamnose to monitor passive transcellular diffusion, changes in gut function and integrity can be monitored and related to the aforementioned model of oral mucositis. The ultimate goal will be to identify those patients at greatest risk of developing bacteraemia or invasive candidiasis soon after starting intensive cytotoxic chemotherapy so that antifungal prophylaxis can be given, and to identify those individuals in whom drug levels are lower because of malabsorption due to intestinal MBI, as this can hamper success (Michallet *et al.* 1998; Prentice & Donnelly 2001).

Conclusions and recommendations

The primary goal of antifungal prophylaxis is to reduce mortality related to invasive candidiasis; but the results are inconclusive. One reason might be simply because the prevalence of invasive candidiasis was too low as fluconazole seemed to be effective only in those studies in which the incidence was higher than 15% (Kanda *et al.* 2000). Hence, to be effective, prophylaxis should be reserved for high-risk groups of patients (Prentice *et al.* 2000). Selection can be based on two criteria, namely *Candida* colonisation of the gut and impaired gut integrity. Colonisation can be determined by twice-weekly surveillance cultures. However, determining impaired gut integrity is still under investigation. An interim solution would be to offer antifungal prophylaxis to the patients mostly likely to develop severe gut MBI such as recipients of either allogenic or autologous HSCT receiving TBI as part of the myeloablative therapy as this is known to be effective (Verfaillie *et al.* 1991; Goodrich *et al.* 1991; Goodman *et al.* 1992; Slavin *et al.* 1995) and also to those receiving their first course of remission-induction therapy for acute myeloid leukaemia with a regimen containing an anthracycline or high-dose cytarabine (Bow *et al.* 1997; Rotstein *et al.* 1999). These two criteria, e.g. *Candida* colonisation and MBI of the gut, can then provide the basis for a management strategy as depicted in Table 3.1.

Table 3.1 Recommendation of antifungal prophylactic therapy risk-targeted towards the presence of colonisation and/or mucosal barrier injury. High-risk group: anthracycline or high-dose cytarabine containing remission-induction therapy or HSCT recipients after TBI-consisting regimens.Other predisposing risk factors are, for example: acute graft versus heart disease, extensive corticosteroid use.

Risk group	*Colonisation*	*Mucosal barrier injury*	*Treatment*
Low	no	no	no
Intermediate	no	yes	no
	yes	no	yes or no*
High	yes	yes	yes

* Depending on other predisposing factors.

References

Bjarnason I, MacPherson A, Hollander D (1995). Intestinal permeability: an overview. *Gastroenterology* **108**, 1566–1581.

Blijlevens NMA, Donnelly JP, De Pauw BE (2000). Mucosal barrier injury: biology, pathology, clinical counterparts and consequences of intensive treatment for haematological malignancy: an overview. *Bone Marrow Transplantation* **25**, 1269–1278.

Bow EJ, Gallant G, Williams GJ *et al.* (1998). Remission induction therapy of untreated acute myeloid leukemia using a non-cytarabine-containing regimen of idarubicin, etoposide, and carboplatin. *Cancer* **83**, 1344–1354.

Bow EJ, Loewen R, Cheang MS, Shore TB, Rubinger M, Schacter B (1997). Cytotoxic therapy-induced D-xylose malabsorption and invasive infection during remission-induction therapy for acute myeloid leukemia in adults. *Journal of Clinical Oncology* **15**, 2254–2261.

Callum JL, Brandwein JM, Sutcliffe SB, Scott JG, Keating A (1991). Influence of total body irradiation on infections after autologous bone marrow transplantation. *Bone Marrow Transplantation* **8**, 245–251.

Daenen S, Muskiet FAJ, Marrink J, Halie MR (1991). Aggressive chemotherapy for acute leukaemia frequently causes intestinal protein leakage. *European Journal of Cancer* **27**, 552–556.

Fegan C, Poynton CH, Whittaker JA (1990). The gut mucosal barrier in bone marrow transplantation. *Bone Marrow Transplantation* **5**, 373–377.

Goodman JL, Winston DJ, Greenfield RA *et al.* (1992). A controlled trial of fluconazole to prevent fungal infections in patients undergoing bone marrow transplantation. *New England Journal of Medicine* **326**, 845–851.

Goodrich JM, Reed EC, Mori M *et al.* (1991). Clinical features and analysis of risk factors for invasive candidal infection after marrow transplantation. *Journal of Infectious Diseases* **164**, 731–740.

Guiot HFI, Fibbe WE, van't Wout JW (1994). Risk factors for fungal infection in patients with malignant hematologic disorders: implications for empirical therapy and prophylaxis. *Clinical Infectious Diseases* **18**, 525–532.

Guiot HFI, Fibbe WE, van't Wout JW (1996). Prevention of invasive candidiasis by fluconazole in patients with malignant hematological disorders and a high grade of candida colonisation. In *Proceedings of the 36th Interscience Conference on Antimicrobial Agents and Chemotherapy, New Orleans*.

Johansson JE, Ekman T (1997). Gastro-intestinal toxicity related to bone marrow transplantation: disruption of the intestinal barrier precedes clinical findings. *Bone Marrow Transplantation* **19**, 921–925.

Kanda Y, Yamamoto R, Chizula A *et al.* (2000). Prophylactic action of oral fluconazole against fungal infection in neutropenic patients. *Cancer* **89**, 1611–1625.

Keefe DM, Cummins AG, Dale BM *et al.* (1997). Effect of high-dose chemotherapy on intestinal permeability in humans. *Clinical Science* **92**, 385–389.

Laverdiere M, Rotstein C, Bow E *et al.* and the Canadian Fluconazole Study Group (2000) Impact of fluconazole prophylaxis on fungal colonization and infection rates in neutropenic patients. *Journal of Antimicrobial Chemotherapy* **46**, 1001–1008.

Martino P, Girmenia C, Venditti M *et al.* (1989). Candida colonization and systemic infection in neutropenic patients. *Cancer* **64**, 2030–2034.

Michallet M, Ppersat F, Kranszhofer N *et al.* (1998). Pharmacokinetics of itraconazole oral solution in allogeneic bone marrow transplant patients receiving total body irradiation *Bone Marrow Transplantation* **21**, 1239–1243.

Micozzi A, Cartoni C, Monaco M, Martino P, Zittoun R, Mandelli F (1996). High incidence of infectious gastrointestinal complications observed in patients with acute myeloid leukemia receiving intensive chemotherapy for first induction of remission. *Supportive Care of Cancer* **4**, 294–297.

Parrilli G, Iaffaioli RV, Martorano M *et al.* (1989). Effects of anthracycline therapy on intestinal absorption in patients with advanced breast cancer. *Cancer Research* **49**, 3689–3691.

Prentice AG, Donnelly JP (2001). Oral antifungals as prophylaxis in haematological malignancy. *Blood Reviews* **15**, 1–8.

Prentice HG, Kibbler CC, Prentice AG (2000). Towards a targeted, risk-based, antifungal strategy in neutropenic patients. *British Journal of Haematology* **110**, 273–284.

Rotstein C, Bow E, Laverdiere M *et al.* and the Canadian Fluconazole Study Group (1999). Randomized placebo-controlled trial of fluconazole prophylaxis for neutropenic cancer patients: benefit based on purpose and intensity of cytotoxic therapy. *Clinical Infectious Diseases* **28**, 340

Samonis G, Gikas A, Anaissie EJ *et al.* (1993). Prospective evaluation of effects of broad-spectrum antibiotics on gastrointestinal yeast colonization of humans. *Antimicrobial Agents and Chemotherapy* **37**, 51–53.

Sandford GR, Merz WG, Wingard JR, Charache P, Saral R (1980). The value of fungal surveillance cultures as predictors of systemic fungal infections. *Journal of Infectious Diseases* **142**, 503–509.

Sandovsky-Losica H, Barr-Nea L, Segal E (1992). Fatal systemic candidiasis of gastrointestinal origine: an experimental model in mice compromised by anti-cancer treatment. *Journal of Medical and Veterinary Mycology* **30**, 219–231.

Sandovsky-Losica H, Segal E (1989). Interaction of *Candida albicans* with murine gastrointestinal mucosa: effect of irradiation on adherence in vitro. *Journal of Medical and Veterinary Mycology* **27**, 345–352.

Sandovsky-Losica H, Segal E (1990). Interaction of *Candida albicans* with murine gastrointestinal mucosa from methotrexate and 5-fluorouracil treated animals: in vitro adhesion and prevention. *Journal of Medical and Veterinary Mycology* **28**, 279–287.

Seipelt G, Hofmann W-K, Martin H *et al.* (1998). Comparison of toxicity and outcome in patients with acute myeloid leukemia treated with high-dose cytosine arabinoside consolidation after induction with a regimen containing idarubicin or daunorubicin. *Annals of Hematology* **76**, 145–151.

Selby P, McElwain TJ, Crofts M, Lopes N, Mundy J (1984). 51Cr-EDTA test for intestinal permeability. *The Lancet* **ii**, 38–39.

Slavin MA, Osborne B, Adams R *et al.* (1995). Efficacy and safety of fluconazole prophylaxis for fungal infections after marrow transplantation – a prospective, randomized, double-blind study. *Journal of Infectious Diseases* **171**, 1545–1552.

Sonis ST (1998). Mucositis as a biological process: a new hypothesis for the development of chemotherapy-induced stomatotoxicity. *Oral Oncology* **34**, 39–43.

Verfaillie C, Weisdorf D, Haake R, Hostetter M, Ramsay NKC, McGlave P (1991). Candida infections in bone marrow transplant recipients. *Bone Marrow Transplantation* **8**, 177–184.

Viscoli C, Girmenia C, Marinus A *et al.* and the Invasive Fungal Infection Group of the EORTC (1999). Candidemia in cancer patients: a prospective, multicenter surveillance study by the Invasive Fungal Infection Group (IFIG) of the European Organization for Research and Treatment of Cancer (EORTC). *Clinical Infectious Diseases* **28**, 1071–1079.

Viscoli C, Paesmans M, Sanz M *et al.* on behalf of the International Antimicrobial Therapy Cooperative Group of the European Organization for Research and Treatment of Cancer (2001). Association between antifungal prophylaxis and rate of documented bacteraemia in febrile neutropenic cancer patients. *Clinical Infectious Diseases* **32**, 1532–1537.

Vlasveld LTH, Zwaan FE, Fibbe WE *et al.* (1991). Neutropenic enterocolitis following treatment with cytosine arabinoside-containing regimens for hematological malignancies. *Annals of Hematology* **62**, 129–134.

Wardley AM, Jayson GC, Swindell R *et al.* (2000). Prospective evaluation of oral mucositis in patients receiving myeloablative conditioning regimens and haematopoietic progenitor rescue. *British Journal of Haematology* **110**, 299.

PART 2

Prophylaxis of SFI

Chapter 4

Systemic fungal infection in the intensive-therapy unit: is there a role for prophylaxis?

Neil Soni and Chris Kibbler

Epidemiology of fungal infection in the surgical patient

Fungal infection in the surgical population has increased over the past two decades. The Centers for Disease Control and Prevention showed that, between 1980 and 1990, *Candida* emerged as the sixth commonest nosocomial pathogen (7.2% of the total) and was the fourth commonest pathogen in nosocomial bloodstream infections. The reasons why this has happened bear closer examination. The patient population is changing, particularly in surgery and in intensive care. Medical management is also evolving and the role of antibiotics, in particular the increasing empirical use of broad-spectrum antibiotics, has probably been important. Nutritional status and the pattern of nutritional regimens may also have a part to play (Rantala 1993). An increasing incidence may also reflect a change in the level of awareness of the problem among medical personnel so that the increase in diagnosis is both real and imagined. This may be particularly relevant because, although fungal infection has always been a source of concern in the immunocompromised, it is only recently that it has come to the fore in the critically ill.

Whether it has always been a major problem in the critically ill is open to debate but it is certainly important now. Reports vary but the incidence of candidaemia in at least one study suggests that it may be more common in the intensive-therapy unit (ITU) than in bone marrow or oncology wards. A report by Giamarellou cites the relative incidence of candidaemia being 25% of cases occurring in surgical intensive-care units (ICUs) versus 25% in bone marrow transplantation units, 20% in medical ICUs, 20% in general medical wards, and 10% in oncology–haematology units (Giamarellou and Antoniadou 1996). The rate at which *Candida* sepsis is reported varies considerably. Diagnosis is still difficult and is probably more common in centres with an interest in the topic; hence epidemiological studies may not necessarily represent the genuine rate. Rantala reported rates of 6.2 per 1000 laparotomies (Rantala *et al.* 1993). In other studies invasive yeast sepsis developed in 17% and 35% of patients (Slotman and Burchard 1987; Eggimann *et al.* 1999). These figures are gleaned not from epidemiology but from the reported incidence of problems in arms of a study. There is clearly a very wide range in the incidence of the problem in the surgical patient. To put it into perspective, in solid organ transplantation the incidence has been reported as 5–50% (Dictar *et al.* 2000). In the bone marrow transplant unit it has been reported as being between 6.7 and 10 infections per 1000 patient days (Berrouane *et al.* 1999). Burns also predispose to nosocomial infection and candidaemia. In burns patients the figures are similar, with a colonisation rate reported as 27%, a superficial infection rate of 21% and a sepsis rate of 12% (Desai *et al.* 1992).

So the problem definitely exists but the magnitude of it is uncertain and relates to the nature of the surgery, the ITU and several other factors. As with other infections the intelligent approach is to know the incidence in the local setting. On the ITU at the Chelsea and Westminster Hospital, London, there are approximately 14 cases of *Candida* sepsis treated per annum (admissions of 500 patients per annum) of which approximately half are confirmed as infection and the others represent a level of anxiety rather than clinical certainty. In the recently completed UK candidaemia study in which nearly 10,000 ITU admissions were included, the incidence of candidaemia in the six sentinel hospitals was 7.4/1000 admissions (Ainscough *et al.* 2000). However, this does not include cases of non-fungaemic sepsis, which are more difficult to diagnose.

It is possible from the literature to list the risk factors that are relevant (Table 4.1) and thereby to identify patients at risk. These include extensive abdominal surgery, and comment has been made on upper gastro-intestinal surgery in particular. In one study 13 out of 37 cases with severe pancreatitis who had operative intervention developed *Candida* sepsis with a very high mortality (Hoerauf *et al.* 1998). Re-operation for infective problems, such as anastamotic leak or intra-abdominal collections, are also notorious, as are patients with underlying malignancy or other immunosuppressive conditions, and patients undergoing transplantation. Ancillary co-factors including central venous catheterisation, parenteral nutrition and prolonged broad spectrum antibiotic therapy are also implicated. There is a high incidence of *Candida* colonisation of central lines and this may be the source of both transient fungaemia and actual invasive infection. It is clearly a problem for the patient who has been hospitalised for a prolonged period (Rantala 1993; Giamarellou and Antoniadou 1996; Dean and Burchard 1998).

Table 4.1 Risk factors

Risk factors
Extensive abdominal surgery
Upper gastro-intestinal surgery
Re-laparotomy for infection/leakage/abscess
Major burns
Nutritional status
Prolonged and broad spectrum antibiotics
Underlying malignancy
Central venous catheterisation
Parenteral nutrition
Liver transplantation
Pancreas transplantation

Given that these risk factors are easily identified in the long-stay surgical patient and that it is likely that colonisation precedes infection, a surgical population at risk can be identified relatively easily.

The other important high risk group in the ITU are the solid-organ transplant patients. Infection rates vary with the type of transplant, being least for renal transplant recipients (approximately 5%) and most for liver transplant recipients (>20%) (Paya 1993). Most infections are caused by *Candida* spp. (approximately 80%) (Wajszczuk *et al.* 1985; Paya 1993). *Pneumocystis carinii* pneumonitis occurs in about 10% of liver, kidney and heart transplant recipients, and in more than 80% of heart–lung and lung transplant recipients not receiving prophylaxis (Gryzan *et al.* 1988). It is closely linked with cytomegalovirus (CMV) disease. Although uncommon, *Cryptococcus neoformans* is the most frequent cause of meningitis in these patients.

The risk factors for fungal infections in liver transplantation include re-transplantation, intra-operative transfusion requirement, emergency status, Roux limb biliary reconstruction, steroid dose, concomitant bacterial infections and antibiotic therapy, and vascular complications (Castaldo *et al.* 1991; Kibbler 1995).

Although it can be seen that most invasive fungal infections encountered in ITU patients are due to *Candida* spp., there is evidence that the prevalence of the different *Candida* species is changing (Patterson 1999). However, this shift away from *Candida albicans* to the other species is not universal and probably reflects the intensity of use of azole antifungal agents and central venous catheters in different populations. In the recently completed UK candidaemia study *Candida albicans* was responsible for 80.6% of cases of fungaemia in ITU patients (Ainscough *et al.* 2000). This contrasted markedly with candidaemia in haematology patients, caused by *C. albicans* in only 27.3%.

Pathogenesis

Traditionally it has always been considered that *Candida* needs a portal of entry into the blood stream, and in the critically ill surgical patient there are multiple possibilities. A stagnant bowel, full of secretions and enteral feed and subjected to broad-spectrum antibiotics, is almost a perfect medium to encourage the overgrowth of *Candida*. Couple this with a less-than-healthy bowel wall and the scene is set for 'translocation'. Elsewhere the surgical wound and any central venous access are obvious portals for invasion.

Animal studies provide some information relating to the colonised gut as a portal of entry of *Candida*. Translocation between the enterocytes, which is the presumed mode of entry of bacteria, is not found in guinea pigs and rats. Instead direct penetration of the cell membrane and movement of *Candida* into the lamina propria causing cell disruption has been shown to occur (Alexander *et al.* 1990). The situation is confused by other studies suggesting guinea pigs are a poor model for *Candida* sepsis (Rietschel *et al.* 1989). The protective mechanisms in the gut wall have been explored and a role for CD4 lymphocytes has been demonstrated in mice. When the gut is heavily colonised with *Candida* it appears that *Candida* antigen induces specific lymphocytes, which appear in the Peyers patches and in the spleen of the mice. This coincides with clearance of *Candida*. So it would appear that this mechanism is intrinsic to the internal defence against *Candida* infection at least in these animal models (Cantorna & Balish 1991).

Attempts have been made to determine whether similar events occur in humans. In one study, susceptible patients, such as those having re-operation, had blood cultures taken but none yielded *Candida*, implying that haematogenous spread intra-operatively was unlikely or at least rare (Rantala 1993).

This has been taken further in a study by McFie who cultured the nasogastric aspirate from surgical patients and then looked at mesenteric lymph nodes during the abdominal procedures. *Candida* was the most frequently isolated organism from nasogastric aspirate but was not found in any lymph nodes. This was in contrast to *E. coli*, which was found in both the nasogastric aspirate and in the mesenteric lymph nodes. This supports the concept of bacterial translocation but fails to implicate this as a mechanism for *Candida* invasion (MacFie *et al.* 1999).

As previously mentioned it has long been postulated that invasion may also take place along catheters or through wounds. The high incidence of *Candida* colonisation on removed central lines would support this contention (Rantala *et al.* 1991).

Although the specific mechanism by which *Candida* invades the blood stream is not proven there is some circumstantial evidence about the preconditions for invasion to take place. There has to be a source and it has been presumed that there must be a significant reservoir of infection. From this has arisen the concept that *Candida* will be found extensively before actual infection and that colonisation will precede invasion. Colonisation does appear to be important. Solomkin noted that increasing colonisation correlated with increasing risk of invasive infection (Solomkin *et al.* 1980). Several investigators have confirmed this and found that colonization almost always precedes infection, usually with a genotypically identical *Candida* spp. strain. Colonisation is, of course, commonly seen in the surgical population. Pittet introduced the concept of using the number of sites colonized and the intensity of colonisation as an index of suspicion of infection and found that the level of colonisation, the corrected candida index (CCI), reached a threshold value about 6 days before actual infection (Pittet *et al.* 1994). This approach is starting to be used in the ITU setting to determine when pre-emptive treatment should start. This concept has been understood for some time in the neutropenic and bone marrow transplant population where it has been proposed as an alternative to prophylaxis (Prentice *et al.* 2000).

It seems that, at least in the surgical setting, *Candida* infection is a problem of long-stay patients. One study refutes this. Rantala reports 8 of 107 patients who developed *Candida* infection in the first post-operative week (Rantala *et al.* 1993).

Candida overgrowth is uncommon in the community and therefore early identification of the organism is an extremely worrying sign as by implication it suggests heavy prior colonisation and thereby a more chronically debilitated patient. Despite this report the concept of colonisation preceding infection is helpful in identifying patients at risk.

Identifying the patient at risk and the magnitude of risk

The work by Pittet enables earlier treatment based on high probability rather than on certainty. The penalty of treating some cases that have extensive colonisation rather than actual infection is almost certainly outweighed by the benefits of earlier intervention. If an understanding of risk factors is coupled with the colonisation index and account taken of the clinical presentation of infection then there is a powerful tool for therapy. This concept could also be applied to the issue of prophylaxis and will be discussed later.

It is possible that other methods may emerge to help quantify risk. It has been suggested that normal phagocytic activity against *C. albicans* is reduced after surgery and after prolonged antibiotics, and this can be demonstrated by flow cytometry. This has potential for identifying patients at risk but the clinical relevance of such a test requires investigation (Tran *et al.* 1997). However, it may be possible to refine the criteria for high-risk patients by using rapid immunological investigations including those of cellular function and humoral components, such as mannose-binding lectins (MBLs).

Early intervention is important. The mortality rate for patients with invasive *Candida* infection post-surgery has been reported as very high. It is probably higher than the mortality associated with most bacterial infections (Rantala 1993). This is for a range of reasons, including the severity of illness of a patient at risk of *Candida* sepsis. It may actually be a marker of severity in its own right. Mortality rates reported vary but are universally high. Crude mortality has been quoted at 50% or exceeding 55% (D'Amelio *et al.* 1995; Giamarellou & Antoniadou 1996). It is possible that improvements in management have resulted in a fall in mortality in recent years. ITU patients were found to have a 30-day mortality of 34% in the UK candidaemia study (Ainscough *et al.* 2000). This level of mortality requires that prophylaxis be considered, whether or not these figures translate to local practice.

Evidence for prophylaxis

Before having this discussion it is essential to define what constitutes prophylaxis. For our purposes it is a management strategy that ideally prevents the acquisition of significant organisms but at minimum reduces the likelihood of proceeding to an infection. The transmission of *Candida* spp. in the ITU setting has been well documented (Burnie *et al.* 1985; Pittet *et al.* 1994) and prevention of acquisition by good infection control practices should be part of the management of these patients.

Transient hand carriage of *Candida* after contact has been shown to occur in more than 60% of cases and subsequent transfer from these hands in more than 30% of cases (Rangel-Frausto 1994). Optimal hand hygiene practices are important, whether or not they are coupled with other prophylactic measures.

There are three different approaches to prophylaxis. The first uses techniques to reduce colonisation and thereby the potential for invasion but without resorting to medication. The second is selective bowel decontamination where *Candida* prophylaxis is part of a much more overarching package of prophylaxis. The third is the use of systemic antifungal agents.

Techniques to reduce *Candida* by alterations in diet and gut function are in their infancy (Heyland *et al.* 1994). As a rule of thumb, in the critically ill it is felt that a mobile active gut is better than a stagnant non-functional gut. It is assumed there is less overgrowth and that the bowel as an organ will remain in a healthier state. In particular the administration of nutrients such as glutamine may be helpful to villous health (Alverdy 1990; Bengmark & Jeppsson 1995; Gianotti *et al.* 1995). This is loosely associated with lower nosocomial infection rates. Therefore efforts are made to keep the bowel active and enteral feeding is encouraged. The argument is made more difficult by the observation that patients with multiple organ failure may have a poorly perfused bowel and that returning the bowel to normal function is not always possible. Unfortunately, these patients are among those with the highest risk of *Candida* infection.

There are few data relating to the influence of enteral feeding on *Candida* colonisation. There are, however, constituents of feed that may influence *Candida* growth. One of these may be yoghurt. *In vitro Streptococcus thermophilus* inhibits *Candida* adherence (Busscher *et al.* 1997). In clinical practice there are several studies that have looked at the impact of dietary yoghurt (containing *Lactobacillus acidophilus*) on vaginal candidiasis with encouraging results for colonisation and, albeit in a very small study, infection (Hilton *et al.* 1992; Shalev *et al.* 1996). If this approach worked it would be highly desirable to use nutritional intervention to reduce the likelihood of colonisation and indeed infection. Currently, the few studies are tantalisingly suggestive, the theoretical argument persuasive, but the data totally inadequate. It should not be dismissed but rather investigated further.

The second approach is selective decontamination of the digestive tract (SDD). Many authors have highlighted the association between antibiotic use and *Candida* overgrowth. It is clear that the general use of antibiotics is associated with fungal infection. It has been observed in neurosurgical patients that the use of prolonged as compared with peri-operative antibiotic prophylaxis for ventricular drainage is associated with increased likelihood of opportunistic infections such as *Candida*. (Poon *et al.* 1998). Other examples abound. Consequently, SDD regimens usually contain an antifungal component in the form of amphotericin B. SDD has been primarily aimed at preventing bacterial infection but there is some evidence for efficacy as antifungal prophylaxis. In a study of 10 liver transplant patients, a single patient developed *Candida* peritonitis but when selective bowel decontamination was discontinued there were three cases seen (van Zeijl *et al.* 1990).

If such antibacterial prophylactic regimens are to be used in a vulnerable population it is essential that antifungals be given, but they should be reserved for very well-defined populations.

The third strategy, the use of antifungal agents to prevent fungal infection, is both the most obvious and the most contentious. The issue is not whether this is effective but rather whether the level of benefit justifies the cost (both real and potential).

The animal models are not necessarily reliable, as is seen with guinea pigs (Rietschel *et al.* 1989). Nevertheless there are studies in mice and rabbits to show the efficacy of fluconazole as a prophylactic agent (Longman *et al.* 1990; Sawyer *et al.* 1995). In humans, most of the information is from well-defined immunocompromised populations, but there are lessons there that may be extrapolated to the surgical population. The agents used in most cases are oral amphotericin B, nystatin and fluconazole. The general consensus is that amphotericin B and the azoles are superior to nystatin (Reents *et al.* 1993). A systematic review on the subject has been published by the Cochrane Collaboration. Accepted studies of nystatin prophylaxis included six trials in leukaemics, one in cancer patients, one in liver transplant recipients, one in AIDS patients and one in surgical and trauma patients. Nystatin performed similarly to placebo. When compared with fluconazole, nystatin was found to be inferior for preventing colonisation and invasive fungal infection. There was no difference in mortality. The conclusion was that nystatin could not be recommended in immunocompromised patients (Gotzsche & Johansen 2003). In a study of cancer patients with neutropenia, the Cochrane database suggests there is only minimal benefit from antifungal agents, but acknowledge limited and heterogenous data (Gotzsche & Johansen 2001). One suggestion from this assessment of prophylaxis in cancer patients is that the use of amphotericin might show benefit. Small numbers were acknowledged, but a number needed to treat of 59 was quoted (Gotzsche & Johansen 2001).

There is variable evidence from specific ITU populations. In 143 liver transplant patients given either nystatin or fluconazole (100 mg daily), *Candida* colonisation occurred in 25% of those on fluconazole and 53% of those on nystatin. *Candida* infection occurred in 13% and 34% of the fluconazole and nystatin groups, respectively. Most of this infection was superficial and the difference in severe infection (2% versus 6%) was not statistically significant, although that probably reflects the small numbers (Lumbreras *et al.* 1996). Nevertheless there is apparent benefit.

A study of 86 liver transplant patients compared liposomal amphotericin B (AmBisome) with placebo. There were no cases of *Candida* infection in the drug group and five invasive *Candida* infections in the placebo group (Tollemar *et al.* 1995). Not all studies have been positive. In a study comparing oral amphotericin and fluconazole (200 mg) the fluconazole was more effective in the treatment of *C. albicans* colonisation, 9/9 versus 6/15, but not other species (Viviani *et al.* 1992). In that study the incidence of fungal colonisation was very high, reported at 67%.

Topical clotrimazole was compared with nystatin by using a different approach and looking at the prevention of oral candidiasis in liver transplant patients. The incidence of colonisation was very low in both groups. These authors suggest either drug is useful to prevent oral problems. Clearly there is considerable disparity in the literature, even of a supposedly homogeneous population such as liver transplantation (Ruskin *et al.* 1992).

Prophylaxis has been widely used in bone marrow transplantation. This is a very different population, where the risk is perceived to be among the highest of any patient population. Fluconazole prophylaxis was compared with placebo in one study. This resulted in a reduction of oropharyngeal colonization by *Candida albicans* and a significant reduction in systemic candidiasis was seen (Goodman *et al.* 1992). In another study, 400 mg fluconazole administered once daily was compared with placebo. There were 10 episodes of systemic infection in 152 patients given fluconazole compared with 26 in 148 given placebo. None of the fungal infections in the fluconazole group were with *Candida albicans*, but there was no significant difference in infections due to non-*albicans* species between the two groups. Fluconazole also reduced superficial infection and the empirical use of amphotericin. Most importantly, mortality at 110 days was reduced in the fluconazole-treated group (Slavin *et al.* 1995).

In pancreatic transplant surgery prophylaxis has been recommended but there are no data (Everett *et al.* 1994). The evidence in the burns population is relatively limited. A study using nystatin suggested a reduction in colonisation; superficial infection and sepsis were all reduced when compared with historical controls (Desai *et al.* 1992).

What does this information bring to the surgical debate? The data are sparse despite the widespread and enthusiastic use of prophylaxis. Such data as exist show a reduction in colonisation with antifungals and suggest that the azoles are superior to nystatin. Nystatin is either equivalent to or better than placebo. The reduction in colonisation is reflected in less superficial infection and less invasive infection. This, however, does not clearly influence mortality. However, the numbers of deaths involved almost certainly preclude definitive analysis of the effect of mortality in these populations.

In surgery there are very few studies. The most important is probably the study by Eggimann. Forty-nine surgical patients with recurrent intestinal perforations or anastamotic leakage were randomised to receive either fluconazole (400 mg/day) or placebo. During surveillance *Candida* was isolated in 15% of the prophylaxis group and 62% of the placebo group. Although there was only one infection in the fluconazole group there were seven cases of *Candida* sepsis in the placebo group.

There was one line-related septic episode in the fluconazole group. This study clearly shows a reduction in both colonisation and in sepsis, albeit with small numbers (Eggimann *et al.* 1999). A previous surgical study from 1987 had a similar message. That study compared ketoconazole and placebo in 57 patients in an ITU. Ketoconazole reduced colonisation significantly and although there was invasive infection in five patients in the placebo group, there was none in the ketoconazole group (Slotman & Burchard 1987).

On the data presented and given the mortality of *Candida* sepsis and the discomfort of superficial infection there is a perceptible benefit in using prophylaxis in certain groups of patients.

Which agent should be used? The argument is that if prophylaxis is to be used then the decision should be to use a therapeutically active agent. The evidence therefore is in favour of fluconazole compared with nystatin.

The argument against the routine use of prophylaxis

Fluconazole is more effective than nystatin, both for reducing colonisation and for reducing the incidence of infection. It has the disadvantage of being an active agent commonly used for treatment and being costly. An additional consideration is that most prophylaxis regimens employ the drug at lower dosages than would normally be used for treatment. This may result in a less than optimal impact of prophylaxis on both colonisation and infection. These lower dosages might also predispose to the development of resistance as well as the emergence of non-*albicans* strains.

In the leukaemic and bone marrow transplantation population there is anxiety about the emergence of more resistant species (Epstein *et al.* 1996). Several authors have commented on changing patterns of organisms. In particular *Candida glabrata* has increased as a problem (Pavese *et al.* 1999; Berrouane *et al.* 1999). It may be possible to prevent or delay the selection of more resistant species by combining azoles with oral amphotericin B (Paterson *et al.* 2001) and this strategy should be explored in other risk groups.

In the management of HIV, the emergence of fluconazole resistance in *Candida albicans* has been seen with persistent colonisation while on prophylaxis. *Candida* was found in 69% of patients receiving fluconazole prophylaxis and 93% of those who did not (Hunter *et al.* 1998). There were 5 patients with fluconazole-resistant *C. albicans* and also 16 patients carrying non-*albicans* yeasts in those who had been exposed to fluconazole. There were only 5 patients with non-*albicans* yeasts in the other group. This suggests that the use of fluconazole can influence subsequent flora. An unusual species, *C. dubliniensis*, which has higher minimal inhibitory concentrations (MICs) to fluconazole (Diz Dios *et al.* 1995; Sullivan & Coleman 1997; Moran *et al.* 1998; Meiller *et al.* 1999) has also been found in this population in association with treatment failure.

There is also evidence of the influence of fluconazole on fungal flora from intensive-care studies. A comparison of two institutions with different fluconazole usage showed a change in flora at the hospital using fluconazole. It was suggested that the widespread use of fluconazole might have been promoting a shift to more resistant species (Gleason *et al.* 1997). Interestingly, most patients treated had negative cultures for *Candida*. In a study of 72 patients treated with fluconazole, 16 had secondary fungal infections, with *C. glabrata* and *C. parapsilosis*. These carried a higher mortality rate than those in patients with a primary fungal infection (Safran & Dawson 1997). A further worrying study in surgical patients found an increased mortality and longer hospital and ICU lengths of stay in the fluconazole-treated patients. The study also implied an alteration in bacterial resistance in those treated. Once again, there may have been a shift in the species of prevalent yeasts, with an increase in non-*albicans* species (Rocco *et al.* 2000).

Conclusions

As with so many areas of critical care, we have inadequate data to make evidence-based decisions. This should not and cannot preclude making decisions. The most obvious conclusion is that more information is required. In the meantime there are areas that can be explored.

Patients who have a high risk for *Candida* infection can be selected using the risk factors identified earlier. The use of low doses of an active agent may have some benefit but carries all the potential risks for resistance and emergence of other species (Flanagan & Barnes 1997). Such practice should be deprecated. Surely the lessons we are still learning in bacteriology in the critically ill should have taught us something.

If a patient is considered to be at very high risk, an active agent should be used. It should be used at a relevant dosage that will result in effective suppression or treatment of infection. This constitutes pre-emptive treatment if used with pre-monitory markers of invasion such as the CCI.

The balance is between the real risk of an infection to an individual, the real efficacy of the prophylaxis in substantially altering that risk, and the real cost to an individual ITU if the flora changes and resistance becomes a problem (Figure 4.1). None of these factors can currently be assessed, but the widespread use of broad-spectrum antibiotics to treat potential problems rather than real ones has been a disaster. There is a real potential for antifungals to follow the same path.

A personal view would be to increase fungal surveillance in high-risk individuals and continually monitor sites of colonisation. In a very high-risk patient (such as a liver transplant recipient), but not in lower-risk groups (such as those undergoing gastro-intestinal tract surgery), a more aggressive approach could be adopted. With progression of numbers of sites colonised and intensity of colonisation, a decision to move to azole prophylaxis would be made (Figure 4.2). In other words, the probability of

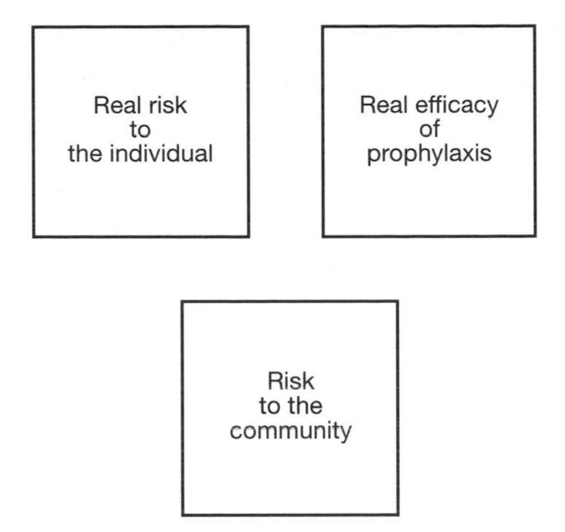

Figure 4.1 Prophylaxis: the balance of risk

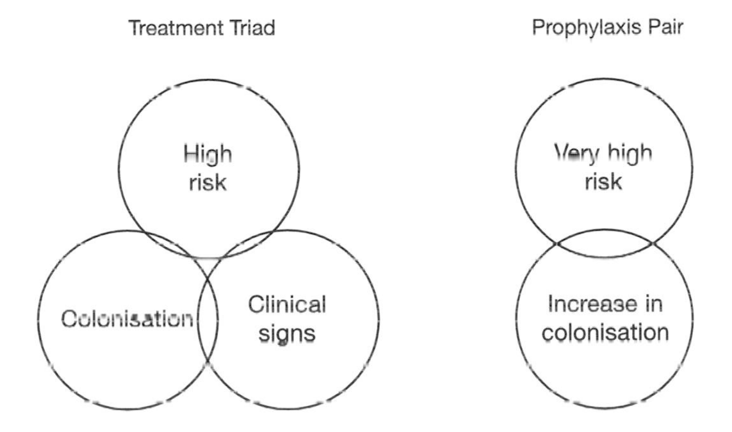

Empirical treatment should be based on a triad of features, whereas prophylaxis should be based on a pair of preconditions.

Figure 4.2 Conditions for instigation of prophylaxis or empirical treatment

developing sepsis can be seen to be increasing in a quantifiable manner; when the probability exceeds a certain threshold prophylaxis is initiated. Prophylaxis in this circumstance would be defined as that adequate to provide effective treatment. This would contrast with the use of empirical treatment in lesser-risk groups, which would commence when the triad of colonisation at mucosal sites, a high-risk patient and clinical features of infection coincide. This strategy essentially reduces the threshold for treatment in the very high-risk groups. It uses the approach described by Pittet and adapts it to very high-risk situations so that treatment is initiated earlier.

It precludes the use of antifungals in patients who are merely high risk and obviates the use of potent agents at sub-therapeutic levels (Giamarellou & Antoniadou 1996). This approach would obviously need study over time to allow analysis of efficacy, toxicity, impact on resistance and cost–benefit.

References

Ainscough S, Barnes R, Gant V *et al.* (2000). Blood stream infections due to *Candida* species in England and Wales: data from the ECMM epidemiological survey of candidaemia in Europe. Abstract P5-032, 6th Congress of the European Confederation of Medical Mycology, Barcelona, 2000.

Alexander JW, Boyce ST *et al.* (1990). The process of microbial translocation. *Annals of Surgery* **212**(4), 496–510.

Alverdy JC (1990). Effects of glutamine-supplemented diets on immunology of the gut. *Journal of Parenteral and Enteral Nutrition* **14** (Suppl. 4), 109s–113s.

Bengmark S and B Jeppsson (1995). Gastrointestinal surface protection and mucosa reconditioning. *Journal of Parenteral and Enteral Nutrition* **19**(5), 410–415.

Berrouane YF, Herwaldt LA *et al.* (1999). Trends in antifungal use and epidemiology of nosocomial yeast infections in a university hospital. *Journal of Clinical Microbiology* **37**(3), 531–537.

Burnie JP, Odds FC, Lee W, Webster C, Williams JD (1985). Outbreak of systemic *Candida albicans* in intensive care unit caused by cross infection. *British Medical Journal* **290**, 746–748.

Busscher HJ, van Hoogmoed CG *et al.* (1997). *Streptococcus thermophilus* and its biosurfactants inhibit adhesion by *Candida* spp. on silicone rubber. *Applied and Environmental Microbiology* **63**(10), 3810–3817.

Cantorna MT, Balish E (1991). Role of CD4+ lymphocytes in resistance to mucosal candidiasis. *Infection and Immunity* **59**(7), 2447–2455.

Castaldo P, Stratta RJ *et al.* (1991). Clinical spectrum of fungal infections after orthotopic liver transplantation. *Archives of Surgery* **126**(2), 149–156.

D'Amelio LF, Wagner B *et al.* (1995). Antibiotic patterns associated with fungal colonization in critically ill surgical patients. *American Surgeon* **61**(12), 1049–1053.

Dean DA, Burchard KW (1998). Surgical perspective on invasive *Candida* infections. *World Journal of Surgery* **22**(2), 127–134.

Desai MH, Rutan RL *et al.* (1992). *Candida* infection with and without nystatin prophylaxis. An 11-year experience with patients with burn injury. *Archives of Surgery* **127**(2), 159–162.

Dictar MO, Maiolo E *et al.* (2000). Mycoses in the transplanted patient. *Medical Mycology* **38** (Suppl 1), 251–258.

Diz Dios PD, Alvarez Alvarez J *et al.* (1995). Fluconazole response patterns in HIV-infected patients with oropharyngeal candidiasis. *Oral Surgery, Oral Medicine, Oral Pathology, Oral Radiology, and Endodontics* **79**(2), 170–174.

Eggimann P, Francioli P *et al.* (1999). Fluconazole prophylaxis prevents intra-abdominal candidiasis in high-risk surgical patients. *Critical Care Medicine* **27**(6), 1066–1072.

Epstein JB, Ransier A *et al.* (1996). Prophylaxis of candidiasis in patients with leukemia and bone marrow transplants. *Oral Surgery, Oral Medicine, Oral Pathology, Oral Radiology, and Endodontics* **81**(3), 291–296.

Everett JE, Wahoff DC *et al.* (1994). Characterization and impact of wound infection after pancreas transplantation. *Archives of Surgery* **129**(12), 1310–1316.

Flanagan PG, Barnes RA (1997). Hazards of inadequate fluconazole dosage to treat deep-seated or systemic *Candida albicans* infection. *Journal of Infection* **35**(3), 295–297.

Giamarellou H, Antoniadou A (1996). Epidemiology, diagnosis, and therapy of fungal infections in surgery. *Infection Control and Hospital Epidemiology* **17**(8), 558–564.

Gianotti L, Alexander JW *et al.* (1995). Oral glutamine decreases bacterial translocation and improves survival in experimental gut-origin sepsis. *Journal of Parenteral and Enteral Nutrition* **19**(1), 69–74.

Gleason TG, May AK *et al.* (1997). Emerging evidence of selection of fluconazole-tolerant fungi in surgical intensive care units. *Archives of Surgery* **132**(11), 1197–1201.

Goodman JL, Winston DJ, Greenfield RA *et al.* (1992). A controlled trial of fluconazole to prevent fungal infections in patients undergoing bone marrow transplantation. *New England Journal of Medicine* **326**(13), 845–851.

Gotzsche PC, Johansen HK (2000). Nystatin prophylaxis and treatment in severely immunodepressed patients (*Cochrane Review*). In: The Cochrane Library. Issue 1, 2003, Oxford: Update Software.

Gotzsche PC, Johansen HK (2000). Routine versus selective antifungal administration for control of fungal infections in patients with cancer (*Cochrane Review*). In: The Cochrane Library. Issue 1, 2003, Oxford: Update Software.

Gryzan S, Paradis IL, Zeevi A *et al.* (1988). Unexpectedly high incidence of *Pneumocystis carinii* infection after lung–heart transplantation. Implications for lung defense and allograft survival. *American Review of Respiratory Diseases* **137**(6), 1268–1274.

Heyland DK, Cook DJ *et al.* (1994). Does the formulation of enteral feeding products influence infectious morbidity and mortality rates in the critically ill patients? A critical review of the evidence. *Critical Care Medicine* **22**(7), 1192–1202.

Hilton E, Isenberg HD *et al.* (1992). Ingestion of yogurt containing *Lactobacillus acidophilus* as prophylaxis for candidal vaginitis. *Annals of Internal Medicine* **116**(5), 353–357.

Hoerauf A, Hammer S *et al.* (1998). Intra-abdominal *Candida* infection during acute necrotizing pancreatitis has a high prevalence and is associated with increased mortality. *Critical Care Medicine* **26**(12), 2010–2015.

Hunter KD, Gibson J *et al.* (1998). Fluconazole-resistant Candida species in the oral flora of fluconazole-exposed HIV-positive patients. *Oral Surgery, Oral Medicine, Oral Pathology, Oral Radiology, and Endodontics* **85**(5), 558–564.

Kibbler CC (1995). Infections in liver transplantation: risk factors and strategies for prevention. *Journal of Hospital Infection* **30** (Suppl.), 209–217.

Longman LP, Hibbert SA *et al.* (1990). Efficacy of fluconazole in prophylaxis and treatment of experimental *Candida* endocarditis. *Reviews of Infectious Diseases* **12** (Suppl 3), S294–S298.

Lumbreras C, Cuervas Mons V *et al.* (1996). Randomized trial of fluconazole versus nystatin for the prophylaxis of *Candida* infection following liver transplantation. *Journal of Infectious Diseases* **174**(3), 583–588.

MacFie J, O'Boyle C *et al.* (1999). Gut origin of sepsis: a prospective study investigating associations between bacterial translocation, gastric microflora, and septic morbidity. *Gut* **45**(2), 223–228.

Meiller TF, Jabra Rizk MA *et al.* (1999). Oral *Candida dubliniensis* as a clinically important species in HIV-seropositive patients in the United States. *Oral Surgery, Oral Medicine, Oral Pathology, Oral Radiology, and Endodontics* **88**(5), 573–580.

Moran GP, Sanglard D *et al.* (1998). Identification and expression of multidrug transporters responsible for fluconazole resistance in *Candida dubliniensis*. *Antimicrobial Agents and Chemotherapy* **42**(7), 1819–1830.

Munoz P, Burillo A *et al.* (2000). Criteria used when initiating antifungal therapy against *Candida* spp. in the intensive care unit. *International Journal of Antimicrobial Agents* **15**(2), 83–90.

Paterson PJ, McWhinney PHM, Potter M, Kibbler CC, Prentice HG (2001). The combination of oral amphotericin B with azoles prevents the emergence of resistant *Candida* species in neutropenic patients. *British Journal of Haematology* **112**, 175–180.

Patterson TF (1999). Role of newer azoles in surgical patients. *Journal of Chemotherapy* **11**(6), 504–512.

Pavese P, Brion JP *et al.* (1999). Epidemiology of fungemia in a university hospital; therapeutic incidence. *Pathologie-biologie (Paris)* **47**(5), 579–583.

Paya CV (1993). Fungal infections in solid-organ transplantation. *Clinical Infectious Diseases* **16**(5), 677–688.

Pittet D, Monod M *et al.* (1994). Candida colonization and subsequent infections in critically ill surgical patients. *Annals of Surgery* **220**(6), 751–758.

Poon WS, Ng S *et al.* (1998). CSF antibiotic prophylaxis for neurosurgical patients with ventriculostomy: a randomised study. *Acta Neurochirurgica (Wien)* (Suppl.) **71**, 146–148.

Prentice HG, Kibbler CC, Prentice AG (2000). Towards a targeted, risk-based, antifungal strategy in neutropenic patients. *British Journal of Haematology* **110**(2), 273–284.

Rangel-Frausto MS, Houston AK, Bale MJ, Fu C, Wenzel RP (1994). An experimental model for study of *Candida* survival and transmission in human volunteers. *European Journal of Clinical Microbiology and Infectious Diseases* **13**, 590–595.

Rantala A (1993). Postoperative candidiasis. *Annales de Chirurgie et Gynaecologie* (Suppl.) **205**, 1–52.

Rantala A, Niinikoski J *et al.* (1991). Pathogenesis of postoperative candidosis: no detectable fungemia during reoperations after abdominal surgery. *Mycoses* **34**(1–2), 47–52.

Rantala A, Niinikoski J *et al.* (1993). Early *Candida* isolations in febrile patients after abdominal surgery. *Scandinavian Journal of Infectious Diseases* **25**(4), 479–485.

Reents S, Goodwin SD *et al.* (1993). Antifungal prophylaxis in immunocompromised hosts. *Annals of Pharmacotherapy* **27**(1), 53–60.

Rietschel P, VanEgmond E *et al.* (1989). The use of ketoconazole in prophylaxis of *Candida* sepsis. *American Surgeon* **55**(7), 462–465.

Rocco TR, Reinert SE *et al.* (2000). Effects of fluconazole administration in critically ill patients, analysis of bacterial and fungal resistance. *Archives of Surgery* **135**(2), 160–165.

Ruskin JD, Wood RP *et al.* (1992). Comparative trial of oral clotrimazole and nystatin for oropharyngeal candidiasis prophylaxis in orthotopic liver transplant patients. *Oral Surgery, Oral Medicine, Oral Pathology* **74**(5), 567–571.

Safran DB, Dawson E (1997). The effect of empiric and prophylactic treatment with fluconazole on yeast isolates in a surgical trauma intensive care unit. *Archives of Surgery* **132**(11), 1184–1188.

Sawyer RG, Adams RB *et al.* (1995). Effectiveness of fluconazole in murine *Candida albicans* and bacterial *C. albicans* peritonitis and abscess formation. *Journal of Medical and Veterinary Mycology* **33**(2), 131–136.

Shalev E, Battino S *et al.* (1996). Ingestion of yogurt containing *Lactobacillus acidophilus* compared with pasteurized yogurt as prophylaxis for recurrent candidal vaginitis and bacterial vaginosis. *Archives of Family Medicine* **5**(10), 593–596.

Slavin MA, Adams B, Levenstein R, Schoch MJ, Feldman, HG *et al.* (1995). Efficacy and safety of fluconazole prophylaxis for fungal infections after marrow transplantation – a prospective, randomized, double-blind study. *Journal of Infectious Diseases* **171**, 1545–1552.

Slotman GJ, Burchard KW, D'Arezzo A, Gann DS (1987). Ketoconazole prevents acute respiratory failure in critically ill surgical patients. *Archives of Surgery* **122**(2), 147–151.

Solomkin JS, Flohr AB, Quie PG, Simmons RL (1980). The role of *Candida* in intraperitoneal infections. *Surgery* **88**(4), 524–530.

Sullivan D, Coleman D (1997). *Candida dubliniensis*: an emerging opportunistic pathogen. *Current Topics in Medical Mycology* **8**(1–2), 15–25.

Tollemar J, Hockerstedt K *et al.* (1995). Liposomal amphotericin B prevents invasive fungal infections in liver transplant recipients. A randomized, placebo-controlled study. *Transplantation* **59**(1), 45–50.

Tran TL, Auger P *et al.* (1997). Perioperative variation in phagocytic activity against *Candida albicans* measured by a flow-cytometric assay in cardiovascular-surgery patients. *Clinical Diagnosis and Laboratory Immunology* **4**(4), 447–451.

van Zeijl JH, Kroes AC *et al.* (1990). Infections after auxiliary partial liver transplantation. Experiences in the first ten patients. *Infection* **18**(3), 146–151.

Viviani MA, Tortorano AM *et al.* (1992). Surveillance and treatment of liver transplant recipients for candidiasis and aspergillosis. *European Journal of Epidemiology* **8**(3), 433–436.

Wajszczuk CP, Dummer JS, Ho M *et al.* (1985). Fungal infections in liver transplant recipients. *Transplantation* **40**(4), 347–353.

Chapter 5

Targeted prophylaxis for systemic fungal infection during treatment for haematological malignancy

DL Turner, A Glasmacher and AG Prentice

Introduction

Targeting prophylaxis implies that some, but not all, anti-fungal drugs may be effective in some, but not all, patients receiving some, but not all, types of treatment for a wide spectrum of haematological malignancies (HMs). The risk of systemic fungal infection (SFI) varies with both the disease and the form of cytotoxic therapy; the stratification of risk has been reviewed in detail (Prentice *et al.* 2000). There are clearly some groups of HM patients at very high risk of SFI, who need prophylaxis, some at very low risk who do not, and a spectrum in between for whom the need for prophylaxis is unclear.

Randomised, controlled trials (RCTs) of these drugs have not always taken such stratification of risk into account. In the trials that have, such as those confined to allogeneic stem cell transplant (SCT) patients, clear-cut results have been obtained, usually in favour of prophylaxis (Goodman *et al.* 1992; Slavin *et al.* 1995; Winston *et al.* 2002). Where RCTs have included a wide range of therapies and HMs, such favourable results have not always been clearly seen (Morgenstern *et al.* 1999; Harousseau *et al.* 2000; Boogaerts *et al.* 2001). Any meta-analysis that includes too great a mixture of targeted and non-targeted studies is likely to reach misleading conclusions, refuting the efficacy of prophylaxis (Gotzsche & Johanssen 1997).

On the other hand, injudicious use of anti-fungal drugs in patients who do not need SFI prophylaxis is likely to lead to premature resistance in yeasts and moulds. Potentially effective prophylaxis could then be lost for those patients who need it most. Fortunately, so far, there has been very little evidence of emerging resistance in SFI organisms in HM patients, unlike the HIV population, but some fungi are intrinsically resistant to some drugs (Johnson *et al.* 1995, 1998). So there is an opportunity to preserve efficacy by restricting or targeting use of current drugs only to high-risk patients or by conducting RCTs of existing and new drugs in high- and intermediate-risk groups only.

Classification of risk has been hampered by diagnostic difficulties described elsewhere in this volume and previously (Chapter 8; Johnson 2001; Barnes 2001; Rogers 2001). These difficulties include the variable extent to which full mycological confirmation is sought and reported by clinicians, a variable application of a range of diagnostic techniques of uncertain sensitivity and specificity by microbiology laboratories and a failure to collect continuously meaningful, national or international fungal, epidemiological data (Denning *et al.* 1998). So targeting of prophylaxis will remain imperfect until these difficulties are resolved. The future impact of the best of the objective laboratory tests (polymerase chain reaction (PCR) and enzyme-linked immunosorbent assay (ELISA)) on prophylaxis will be interesting to observe (Hebart *et al.* 2000; Maertens *et al.* 2001). At present, it is unclear how results of these tests can be used to start, continue or stop prophylaxis in HM patients at high and intermediate risk. Perhaps the recent statement on levels of diagnostic certainty (Ascioglu *et al.* 2002) will impose a definition of definite infection, at least in RCTs if not in clinical practice.

The third and arguably most important aspect of targeting is the choice of drug. Effective SFI prophylaxis requires accurate assessment of *in vitro* and *in vivo* efficacy and *in vivo* utility and toxicity of each drug. There is an abundance of such data for many drugs, but the past development of studies appears haphazard. There has been a frequent failure to pursue uniform, sequential, structured programmes of investigation from laboratory *in vitro* studies of maximum inhibitory concentrations (MICs) through to adequately powered, risk-stratified and double-blind RCTs of new drugs versus 'known best' drugs or placebo. Included in this progressive approach should be the essential, intermediate pharmacokinetic (PK) studies in the patient population to be targeted in RCTs and clinical practice. Too often, such studies have followed the RCT, on the assumption that PK profiles from normal subjects apply to HM patients. Usually they do not for several reasons such as poor nutritional state, end-organ dysfunction (particularly hepatic, but also renal), concomitant infection and concomitant, highly toxic therapy, some of which will interact directly and indirectly with the prophylactic drug.

So the summary profile of the ideal anti-fungal prophylactic drug would be efficacy over the complete range of yeasts and fungi causing SFIs in HM patients. Adequate bioavailability should mean that trough or pre-dose concentrations (C_{min}) are at least as high as *in vitro* MICs. Such bioavailability should be achievable by oral (PO) or intravenous (IV) administration. Toxicity should not compromise efficacy or utility, or lead to additional problems for patients and their physicians who already have enough to contend with. These are tough targets and few if any drugs achieve them all. In the previous volume of this series, the extent to which the frequently used anti-fungal drugs measured up to these targets was reviewed (Prentice 2001). That review is now summarised with additional evidence for existing and new drugs.

Polyenes

Both nystatin and amphotericin B have excellent activity against almost the full spectrum of yeasts and moulds causing SFIs in HM patients. However, neither achieves more than 5% systemic bioavailability if given PO. This disadvantage may be useful clinically as PO polyenes may reduce candidal gut colonisation and therefore SFIs (Cole *et al.* 1996). This would be particularly relevant in combination with the highly absorbed PO triazoles, which may not reach the large gut in sufficient concentration to deal with *Candida* spp. (Odds *et al.* 1989; Rosenberg-Arska *et al.* 1991; Prentice *et al.* 1994).

Conventional nystatin is unsuitable for IV use. A liposomal preparation is undergoing clinical trials, but there are insufficient data to judge it against the above criteria for effective prophylaxis.

There is good correlation between *in vitro* MICs and clinical outcome for both *Candida* and *Aspergillus* spp. for IV amphotericin B (Bryce *et al.* 1992; Lass-Florl *et al.* 1998); the higher the dose, the better the clinical outcome. Despite this, one small RCT has shown a significant reduction in SFI in a high-risk group of allogeneic SCT patients given a very low dose (5–10 mg daily) IV (O'Donnell *et al.* 1994). The well-known toxicity of this drug when given IV (Gallis *et al.* 1990) certainly limits its use in prophylaxis.

Liposomal amphotericin B (Ambisome) IV reduced these toxicities significantly (Prentice *et al.* 1997) making this potent anti-fungal drug a candidate for effective prophylaxis. Again only one small (double-blind) RCT of prophylaxis in high-risk allogeneic SCT patients showed a significant reduction in SFI with Ambisome (Tollemar *et al.* 1993). This was not confirmed in a subsequent, larger RCT (Kelsey *et al.* 1999). Of greater interest are the results of two, large, empirical therapy trials of IV Ambisome in suspected SFI in a wide range of HM (and solid tumour) patients and types of therapy (including SCT) (Walsh *et al.* 1999, 2002). In both these studies the incidence rate of breakthrough, proven SFI, after the start of Ambisome (a clinical surrogate for prophylaxis), was impressively low and, in the first study, significantly lower compared with IV conventional amphotericin B. In the second study the rate was not quite so impressively low in the high-risk patients. However, these results imply that IV Ambisome may be a very effective anti-fungal, prophylactic drug, but only at high dose and therefore at great expense. In the second study (Walsh *et al.* 2002), Ambisome was significantly out-performed by voriconazole, a new triazole, which produced a lower incidence rate of proven, breakthrough SFI, particularly in the high-risk group of patients (see below).

Triazoles

This group of drugs (fluconazole, itraconazole, voriconazole and posaconazole) has very varied *in vitro* and clinical activity against yeasts and moulds, PK and bioavailability profiles, modes of delivery and toxicities. It is therefore inappropriate to think of them as having a class action in SFI prophylaxis, and even a meta-analysis of HM trials of triazoles alone may not be sufficiently powerful or targeted to detect efficacy (Bow *et al.* 1999). All these triazoles are metabolised by cytochrome p450 which means that they all pose drug interaction problems, but again to varying degrees.

Fluconazole

Fluconazole has been the most widely used of this group, despite the fact that it is fully active against only *C. albicans* and *C. tropicalis*, variably active against *C. glabrata* and inactive again *C. krusei* and *Aspergillus* spp. (Anaissie *et al.* 1995; Rex *et al.* 1997). Given PO it is over 90% bioavailable systemically (Sugar *et al.* 1993) and PK profiles are the same for PO and IV administration with a low volume of distribution and rapid achievement of C_{min} equivalent to MICs for *C. albicans* even in allogeneic SCT patients (El Yazigi *et al.* 1997). RCTs have confirmed *in vitro* and PK studies in showing that fluconazole reduces significantly only *C. albicans* SFIs in high-risk SCT patients (Goodman *et al.* 1992; Slavin *et al.* 1995), but not in patients given chemotherapy for HM. A meta-analysis of sixteen RCTs confirmed that fungal-related deaths were 0–8.7% in the fluconazole group and 0–12.8% in the control group (odds ratio (OR) = 0.45, 95% confidence interval (CI) = 0.29–0.72), but that this beneficial effect arose from bone marrow transplantation (BMT) trials only. Prophylactic fluconazole was not effective in reducing fungal-related death or in reducing proven, systemic fungal infections in trials of non-BMT patients only (OR = 0.91, 95% CI = 0.30–2.82 and OR = 0.85, 95% CI = 0.47–1.55) (Kanda *et al.* 2000). However, fluconazole was very effective in reducing superficial fungal infections (OR = 0.44, 95% CI = 0.24–0.80), even when it was given in lower doses (50–200 mg per day). There was no increase in proven, systemic infection of fluconazole-resistant fungi, although colonisation by those fungi increased. In five relatively small trials with incidence rates of SFI greater than 15% in the control (inactive) arm, meta-analysis suggested that fluconazole was effective in reducing such infections (OR = 0.23, 95% CI = 0.15–0.36), but this is likely to be due to an anti-*C. albicans* effect in heavily immunosuppressed patients.

Itraconazole

Itraconazole has *in vitro* activity over a wide spectrum of *C. albicans* and non-*albicans* spp. (Rex *et al.* 1997) and, more importantly, has activity against *Aspergillus* spp. equivalent to amphotericin B (Dupont & Druchet 1987; Van Cutsem *et al.* 1987). The problem of variable and poor absorption with the PO capsule form (Bradford *et al.* 1991) was overcome by the introduction of a cyclodextrin solution which achieves C_{min} likely to be effective against *Candida* and *Aspergillus* spp. within 14 days of the start of PO administration, even in allogeneic SCT patients (Boogaerts *et al.* 1989; Prentice *et al.* 1995; Michallet *et al.* 1998; Glasmacher *et al.* 2001). The parent drug is hydroxylated to an equally active form which accumulates at twice the rate of itraconazole and both forms achieve large volumes of distribution, terminal saturation kinetics in blood and tissues and prolonged wash-out times. A retrospective, multivariate logistic regression analysis of neutropenic patients with haematological malignancies and itraconazole prophylaxis identified a trough concentration of 500 ng/ml itraconazole at the end of the first week of prophylaxis as an independent protective factor for invasive fungal infections whereas lower concentrations did not protect against these infections (Glasmacher *et al.* 1999a, 2000). Therefore, it may be important to use loading dose regimens that can easily achieve these concentrations (Glasmacher *et al.* 1999b).

There have been nine RCTs of this drug as SFI prophylaxis in HM, four using capsules (Vreudgenhil *et al.* 1993; Annaloro *et al.* 1995; Huijgens *et al.* 1999; Nucci *et al.* 2000) and five using the solution (Menichetti *et al.* 1999; Morgenstern *et al.* 1999; Harousseau *et al.* 2000; Boogaerts *et al.* 2001; Winston *et al.* 2002). All nine have been subjected to meta-analysis which shows a significant reduction with itraconazole in SFI overall (OR = 0.58, 95% CI = 0.39–0.84, $p = 0.004$), in yeast SFI (OR = 0.42, 95% CI = 0.23–0.77, $p = 0.005$) and in SFI deaths (OR = 0.55, 95% CI = 0.34–0.90, $p = 0.02$) (Glasmacher *et al.* 2001). In sub-group analysis, predictably, this statistical significance was found only in the group of solution studies and not in those using capsules. In the solution sub-group analysis, *Aspergillus* SFI were also reduced by itraconazole (OR = 0.46, 95% CI = 0.23–0.92, $p = 0.03$).

In the last of these solution trials (Winston *et al.* 2002), itraconazole prophylaxis started with a 14-day IV infusion followed by oral administration and a switch back to IV itraconazole was allowed if PO intake failed for any reason. This trial, conducted exclusively in allogeneic SCT patients has shown a very clear reduction in *Aspergillus* SFI (3/71 versus 8/67, OR = 0.35, 95% CI = 0.10–1.20, $p = 0.094$). This illustrates the points made above about targeting the drug to the pathogen in the appropriate high-risk population and ensuring delivery of bioavailability (switch from PO to IV).

Failure of PO intake due to nausea is itraconazole's main drawback (apart from diarrhoea and hypokalaemia) (Morgenstern *et al.* 1999), but IV administration circumvents this and PK studies indicate a need for cautious dosing with IV administration because of the combined high levels of itraconazole and hydroxyitraconazole achieved by this route (Prentice *et al.* 2000). This is particularly important because of unpredictable and idiosyncratic interaction with cyclosporin (Kramer *et al.* 1997). However, in practice, cyclosporin levels are monitored frequently, this interaction is detected early and is managed effectively by reducing the cyclosporin dose to one third. It is best avoided in regimens containing vincristine because of its ability to exaggerate the neurotoxicity of this alkaloid (Bohme *et al.* 1995). Finally, there is a very rare reported association with congestive cardiac failure due to a negative inotropic effect of itraconazole (Ahmad *et al.* 2001; CMS/MCA 2001).

Voriconazole

Voriconazole is a new broad-spectrum triazole with a similar mechanism of action to the other triazoles. *In vitro* testing has shown that voriconazole is active against *Aspergillus* and *Candida* spp. at an MIC of 0.25–8 μg/ml. It has fungicidal activity against a wide range of agents including *Aspergillus* spp. and *Fusarium* spp. and has potent *in vitro* activity against *Candida* spp. including non-*albicans* spp. which are resistant to fluconazole. PK data from healthy volunteer studies show that twice-daily dosing is appropriate after an initial loading dose and steady state is reached within 24 hours. With rapid oral absorption, maximum concentrations are reached in less than 2 hours and bioavailability is 90%, although food decreases the absorption. The recommended oral loading is 400 mg b.d. on day 1 followed by 200 mg b.d. maintenance. The IV equivalent is 6 mg/kg b.d. loading with 3 mg/kg b.d. subsequently. Voriconazole is metabolised, as are other triazoles, by human cytochrome P450, and metabolites do not have anti-fungal activity. Its clearance is largely hepatic. There are potential interactions as with other triazoles, such as with cyclosporin and vinca akaloids. Data for patients undergoing chemotherapy and bone marrow transplantation are not yet available where bioavailability may differ because of the factors described above. Such studies are now at the stage of design and will hopefully be completed in advance of any RCTs of SFI prophylaxis in HM.

So far, the evidence of clinical efficacy of this drug has been encouraging. In an RCT of voriconazole versus Ambisome in the empirical treatment of suspected SFI in 837 neutropenic patients with persistent fever there was a slightly inferior response with voriconazole, although this difference was not significant (Walsh *et al.* 2002). Of greater interest is the difference in proven breakthrough SFI during this empirical therapy (a clinical surrogate for prophylaxis). This study was not confined to patients with HM, but in those HM patients at high risk of SFI there was a significantly lower rate of proven, breakthrough SFI with voriconazole, whether the patients had been given systemically active prophylaxis before treatment randomisation or not (1.7% versus 9.5%, respectively, $p = 0.003$ for both). This significance was not seen in patients with only a moderate risk of SFI. This result merits a formal, confirmatory prophylaxis study. About 20% of patients experience transient and minor visual hallucinations, but there are few other significant side-effects.

Posaconazole

Posaconazole is another new triazole which also has activity against a wide variety of yeasts and fungi including strains of *Candida* that are resistant to fluconazole. The *in vitro* MIC for *Aspergillus* ranges from less than 0.002 to 0.5 μg/ml and for *Candida* spp. less than 0.004 to16 mg/ml (Cacciapuoti 2000).

In healthy volunteers, after a single dose the C_{max} ranges from 113 to 1320 ng/ml increasing with doses up to a maximum of 800 mg. Posaconazole is slowly orally absorbed and the mean time to maximum concentration is 5 hours with a half life of

25 hours. It is eliminated in a dose-independent fashion with a large volume of distribution, indicating that it is distributed extensively in tissues. Multiple dosing studies in normal volunteers who received up to 800 mg/day for 24 days produced similar half-lives and volumes of distribution and mean trough concentrations were reached by day 10.

Posaconazole, like other azoles, is metabolised by cytochrome P450 and caution is required with concomitant administration of such other drugs. In a phase 1 safety study no dose-related increase in side-effects was observed and the most frequent adverse events were non-specific dizziness and fatigue. Similarly, phase II and III studies in HIV-positive patients with candidosis showed no obvious drug-related adverse reactions. Trough pre-dose concentrations exceeded 400 ng/ml in most patients with invasive fungal infections treated with 800 mg/day.

Bioavailability is increased with high fat meals, which is of concern in patients with HM who often have poor food intake. The oral suspension has a greater bioavailability (35%) than the tablet formulation and may be useful for this group. There is no IV formulation at present, which may hamper its use as prophylaxis in patients who are unable to tolerate PO medication. Further pharmacokinetic and efficacy trials may be underway for both the treatment of and prophylaxis against SFI.

Caspofungin

Caspofungin is the first of a new class of anti-fungal agents, the glucan synthetase inhibitors, which target β (1,3)-D-glucan, an integral part of the fungal cell wall. Caspofungin has a half-life of 10 hours and is extensively bound to albumin. It is metabolised by hydrolysis and acetylation. In patients with mild renal impairment there is no increase in plasma concentration, but patients with moderate or severe renal failure experience an increase in the plasma concentrations after a single-dose infusion. However, in patients with invasive aspergillosis given multiple daily dosing, no significant increase in trough levels was observed with any degree of renal impairment, so dosage adjustment is not required in renal failure. Patients with moderate hepatic impairment have significantly increased bioavailability compared with normal controls, therefore dosage adjustment is required. Caspofungin shows activity both *in vitro* and *in vivo* against a wide range of yeasts and fungi including *Aspergillus* and *Candida* spp. and is licensed for use in refractory *Aspergillus* infections or for those patients intolerant of other therapies (Keating *et al.* 2001). Standardised susceptibility testing methods have not yet been established and results do not correlate so far with clinical outcome. Caspofungin does not interact with other drugs in the cytochrome P450 system or other anti-fungal drugs. The glucan synthetase inhibitors act only against the fungal cell wall and not against the mammalian cell thus potentially reducing toxicity.

As yet there are limited data about the use of this drug in SFI and no data on prophylaxis. In a non-comparative study of 54 patients with invasive aspergillosis who failed to respond to or did not tolerate other anti-fungal agents, complete or partial responses were seen in 41% of patients who were treated with Caspofungin for greater than 7 days (70 mg IV as a 1 hour infusion as loading dose and then subsequently 50 mg IV daily). Clinical adverse effects occurred in 4% of patients and these were mainly fever, flushing and infusional venous complications and adverse laboratory events were proteinuria and eosinophilia (Maertens *et al.* 2000). A phase 2 trial comparing Caspofungin and Amphotericin B in locally invasive *Candida* infections showed a superior tolerability and safety profile with similar efficacy (Arathoon *et al.* 2002). This new class of drugs is promising as it is clinically active against a wide variety of fungi and has relatively few side-effects, although no oral compound is available. Randomised controlled trials in patients with HM are needed to compare Caspofungin with more standard drugs such as Amphotericin B and the triazoles in both treatment and prophylactic settings. However, the utility of this drug will always be limited for prophylaxis. Its molecular size and complexity make it highly unlikely that an oral form will ever be available. Orally administered, systemically active prophylaxis may be needed for post-transplant patients who are at very high risk from community-acquired SFI (*Aspergillus* spp. in particular) up to 1 year after conditioning (Jantunen *et al.* 1997).

Summary

Taking this demanding, targeting approach to determining the ability of an anti-fungal drug to provide effective SFI prophylaxis leads one to an inescapable conclusion. Despite the limitations of its toxicity and palatability, itraconazole is still the only drug that comes close to meeting all the targets on current evidence. Further studies of voriconazole may reveal that it shares or betters itraconazole's record. But it remains uncertain whether RCTs of voriconazole will be targeted appropriately or will wait for the results of PK studies.

References

Ahmad S, Singer S, Leissa B (2001). Congestive heart failure associated with itraconazole. *Lancet* **357** (9270), 1766–1767.

Anaissie EJ, Kontoyiannis DP, Huls C *et al.* (1995). Safety, plasma concentrations, and efficacy of high dose fluconazole in invasive mould infections. *Journal of Infectious Diseases* **172**, 599–602.

Annaloro C, Oriani A, Taglliaferri E *et al.* (1995). Efficacy of different prophylactic anti-fungal regimes in bone marrow transplantation. *Haematologica* **80**(6), 512–517.

Arathoon EG, Gobuzzo E, Nonega LM, Berman RS, DiNubile MJ, Sable CA (2002). Randomized, double-blind, multicenter study of caspofungin versus amphotericin B for treatment of oropharyngeal and esophageal candidiases. *Antimicrobial Agents and Chemotherapy* **46**(2), 451–457.

Ascioglu S, Rex J, de Pauw B *et al.* (2002). Defining opportunistic invasive fungal infections in immunocompromised patients with cancer and haemopoietic stem cell transplants. *Clinical Infectious Diseases* **34**, 7–14.

Barnes RA (2001). Environmental factors in the determination of risk. In *The Effective Prevention and Management of Systemic Fungal Infection in Haematological Malignancy* (eds Prentice A, Rogers T and Miles A), pp. 23–30. Aesculapius Medical Press, London, UK.

Bohme A, Ganser A, Hoelzer D (1995). Aggravation of vincristine-induced neurotoxicity by itraconazole in the treatment of adult ALL. *Annals of Haematology* **71**, 311–312.

Boogaerts M, Winston DJ, Bow EJ *et al.* (2001). Intravenous and oral itraconazole versus intravenous amphotericin B deoxycholate as empirical therapy for persistent fever in neutropenic patients with cancer who are receiving broad-spectrum intravenous antibacterial therapy: a randomised controlled trial. *Annals of Internal Medicine* **135**, 412–422.

Boogaerts MA, Verhoef GE, Zachee P *et al.* (1989). Anti-fungal prophylaxis with itraconazole in prolonged neutropenia: correlation with plasma levels. *Mycoses* **32** (Suppl.1), 103–108.

Bow EJ, Laverdiere M, Lussier N *et al.* (1999). Anti-fungal prophylaxis in neutropenic cancer patients – a meta-analysis of randomised controlled trials. *Blood* **94**, 339a.

Bradford CR, Prentice AG, Warnock D, Copplestone JA (1991). Comparison of the multiple dose pharmacokinetics of two formulations of itraconazole during remission induction for acute myelobastic leukaemia. *Journal of Antimicrobial Chemotherapy* **28**, 55–60.

Bryce EA, Roberts FJ, Sekhon AS, Coldman AJ (1992). Yeast in blood cultures. Evaluation of factors influencing outcome. *Diagnostic Microbiology and Infectious Disease* **15**, 233–237.

Cacciapuoti A, Loebenberg D, Corcoran E *et al.* (2000). In vitro and in vivo activities of SCH 5692 (posaconazole), a triazole antifungal agent, against *Aspergillus* and *Candida*. *Antimicrobial Agents Chemotherapy* **44**(8), 2017–2022.

CSM (MCA) (2001). Cardiodepressant effect of Itraconazole (Sporanox). *Current Problems in Pharmacovigilance* **21**, 9.

Cole GT, Halawa AA, Annaise EJ (1996). The role of the gastrointestinal tract in hematogenous candidiasis: from the laboratory to the bedside. *Clinical Infectious Diseases* **22**, S73–S88.

Denning DW, Marinus A, Cohen J *et al.* (1998). An EORTC multi-centre prospective survey of invasive *Aspergillus* in haematological patients: diagnosis and therapeutic outcome. *Journal of Infection* **37**, 173–180.

Dupont B, Druchet E (1987). Early experience with itraconazole *in vitro* and in patients: pharmacokinetic studies and clinical results. *Reviews in Infectious Diseases* **9** (Suppl.1), S71–S76.

El Yazigi A, Ellis M, Ernst P *et al.* (1997). Effect of repeated dosing on the pharmacokinetics of oral fluconazole in bone marrow transplant patients. *Journal of Clinical Pharmacology* **37**, 1031–1037.

Gallis HA, Drew RH, Pickard WW (1990). Amphotericin B: 30 years of clinical experience. *Reviews in Infectious Diseases* **12**, 308–329.

Glasmacher A, Hahn C, Leutner C, Molitor E, Wardelmann E, Losem C, Sauerbruch T, Marklein G, Schmidt-Wolf, IGH (1999a). Breakthrough invasive fungal infections in neutropenic patients after prophylaxis with itraconazole. *Mycoses* **42**, 443–451.

Glasmacher A, Hahn C, Molitor E, Sauerbruch T, Marklein G, Schmidt-Wolf IGH (1999b). Itraconazole trough concentrations in antifungal prophylaxis with six different dosing regimens using hydroxy β-propyl-cyclodextrin oral solution or coated pellet capsules. *Mycoses* **42**, 591–600.

Glasmacher A, Hahn C, Molitor E, Sauerbruch T, Marklein G, Schmidt-Wolf IGH (2000). Definition of an itraconazole target concentration for antifungal prophylaxis. In *Proceedings of the Interscience Conference on Antimicrobial Agents and Chemotherapy*, Toronto, Canada; vol. 40, p. 663. American Society of Microbiology, Washington DC.

Glasmacher A, Hahn C, Molitor E, Marklein G, Schmidt-Wolf IGH (2001). Itraconazole for antifungal prophylaxis in neutropenic patients: A meta-analysis of 2181 patients. *Proceedings of the Interscience Conference on Antimicrobial Agents and Chemotherapy*, Toronto, Canada; vol. 40, p. 378. American Society of Microbiology, Washington DC.

Glasmacher A, Djulbegovic B, Prentice A, Hahn C, Schmidt-Wolf IGH (2002). Meta-analysis of itraconazole antifungal prophylaxis trials reveals a dose–response effect for the prevention of invasive fungal infections, including *Aspergillus*, in neutropenic patients. *Blood* **100**(11, part1), 216a.

Goodman JL, Winston DJ, Greenfield RA *et al.* (1992). A controlled trial of fluconazole to prevent fungal infections in patients undergoing bone marrow transplantation. *New England Journal of Medicine* **326**, 845–851.

Gotzsche PC and Johanssen HK (1997). Meta-analysis of prophylactic or empirical antifungal treatment versus placebo or no treatment in patients with cancer complicated by neutropenia. *British Medical Journal* **314**, 1238–1244.

Harousseau JL, Dekker AW, Stamatoullas-Bastard A *et al.* (2000). Itraconazole oral solution for primary prophylaxis of fungal infections in patients with haematological malignancy and profound neutropenia: a randomised, double-blind, placebo, multicentre trial comparing itraconazole and amphotericin B. *Antimicrobial Agents and Chemotherapy* **44**, 1887–1893.

Hebart H, Loeffler J, Meisner C *et al.* (2000). Early detection of *Aspergillus* infection after allogeneic stem cell transplantation by polymerase chain reaction screening. *Journal of Infectious Diseases* **181**, 1713–1719.

Huijgens PC, Simons-Smit AM, van Loenen AC *et al.* (1999). Fluconazole versus itraconazole for the prevention of fungal infections in haemato-oncology. *Journal of Clinical Pathology* **52**(5), 376–380.

Jantunen E, Ruutu P, Niskanen L *et al.* (1997). Incidence and risk factors for invasive fungal infections in allogeneic BMT recipients. *Bone Marrow Transplantation* **19**, 801–808.

Johnson EM (2001). Epidemiological aspects of systemic fungal infection: incidence, prevalence and analysis of trends. In *The Effective Prevention and Management of Systemic Fungal Infection in Haematological Malignancy* (eds Prentice A, Rogers T and Miles A), pp. 3–21. Aesculapius Medical Press, London, UK.

Johnson EM, Davey KG, Szekely A, Warnock DW (1995). Itraconazole susceptibilities of fluconazole susceptible and resistant isolates of five *Candida* species. *Journal of Antimicrobial Chemotherapy* **36**, 787–793.

Johnson EM, Szekely A, Warnock DW (1998). *In-vitro* activity of voriconazole, itraconazole and amphotericin B against filamentous fungi. *Journal of Antimicrobial Chemotherapy* **42**, 741–745.

Kanda Y, Yamamoto R, Chizuka A *et al* (2000). Prophylactic action of oral fluconazole against fungal infection in neutropenic patients. A meta-analysis of 16 randomized, controlled trials. *Cancer* **89**, 1611–1625.

Keating GM and Jarvis B (2001). Caspofungin. *Drugs* **61**(8), 1121–1129.

Kelsey SM, Goldman JM, McCann S *et al.* (1999). Liposomal amphoteracin B (AmBisome) in the prophylaxis of fungal infections in neutropenic patients: a randomised, double blind, placebo-controlled study. *Bone Marrow Transplantation* **23**, 163–168.

Kramer MR, Merin G, Rudis E *et al.* (1997). Dose adjustment and cost of itraconazole prophylaxis in lung transplant recipients receiving cyclosporin and tacrolimus (FK506). *Transplant Proceedings* **29**, 2657–2659.

Lass-Flörl C, Kofler G, Kropshofer G *et al.* (1998). *In-vitro* testing of susceptibility to amphotericin B is a reliable predictor of outcome in invasive aspergillosis. *Journal of Antimicrobial Chemotherapy* **42**, 497–502.

Maertens J, Raad I, Sable CA *et al.* (2000). Multi-centre, non-comparative study to evaluate safety and efficacy of Caspofungin in adults with invasive aspergillosis refractory or intolerant to amphoteracin B (AMB), AMB lipid formulations or azoles. 40th *Interscience Conference on Antimicrobial Agents and Chemotherapy*; Toronto.

Maertens J, Verhaegen J, Lagrou K *et al.* (2001). Screening for circulating galactomannan as a non-invasive diagnostic tool for invasive aspergillosis in prolonged neutropenia patients and stem cell transplantation recipients: a prospective validation. *Blood* **97**(6), 1604–1610.

Menichetti F, Del Favero A, Martino P *et al.* (1999). Itraconazole oral solution as prophylaxis for fungal infections in neutropenic patients with hematologic malignancies: a randomised, placebo-controlled, double blind, multicentre trial. GIMEMA infection programme. Groupo Italiano Malattie Ematologische del Alto. *Clinical Infectious Diseases* **28**, 250–255.

Michallet M, Persat F, Kranzhofer N *et al.* (1998). Pharmokinetics of itraconazole oral solution in allogeneic bone marrow transplant patients receiving total body irradiation. *Bone Marrow Transplantation* **21**, 1239–1243.

Morgenstern GR, Prentice AG, Prentice HG *et al.* (1999). A randomised controlled trial of itraconazole versus fluconazole for the prevention of fungal infections in patients with haematological malignancies. *British Journal of Haematology* **105**, 901–911.

Nucci M, Biasoli I, Akiti T *et al.* (2000). A double blind, randomised, placebo controlled trial of itraconazole capsules as antifungal prophylaxis for neutropenic patients. *Clinical Infectious Diseases* **30**(2), 300–305.

O'Donnell MR, Schmidt GM, Tegtmeier BR *et al.* (1994). Prediction of systemic fungal infection in allogeneic marrow recipients: impact of amphotericin prophylaxis in high-risk patients. *Journal of Clinical Oncology* **12**, 827–834.

Odds FC, Kibbler CC Walker E *et al.* (1989). Carriage of *Candida* species and *C. albicans* biotypes in patients undergoing chemotherapy or bone marrow transplantation for haematological disease. *Journal of Clinical Pathology* **42**, 1259–1266.

Prentice AG (2001). Evidence for effective prophylaxis of infection: a review of pharmacokinetic and trial data. In *The Effective Prevention and Management of Systemic Fungal Infection in Haematological Malignancy* (eds Prentice A, Rogers T and Miles A), pp. 51–64. Aesculapius Medical Press, London, UK.

Prentice AG, Copplestone JA, Hamon MD *et al.* (2000). Intravenous itraconazole can replace oral solution in aspergillosis prophylaxis: pharmacokinetic data from patients treated for haematological malignancy. *British Journal of Haematology* 2000; **108**(1), 68a.

Prentice HG, Kibbler CC, Prentice AG (2000). Towards a targeted, risk-based, anti-fungal strategy in neutropenic patients. *British Journal of Haematology* **110**, 273–284.

Prentice HG, Hann I, Herbrecht R *et al.* (1997). A randomised comparison of liposomal versus conventional amphotericin B for treatment of pyrexia of unknown origin in neutropenic patients. *British Journal of Haematology* **98**(3), 711–718.

Prentice AG, Warnock DW, Johnson SA *et al.* (1995). Multiple dose pharmacokinetics of an oral solution of itraconazole in patients receiving chemotherapy for acute myeloid leukaemia. *Journal of Antimicrobial Chemotherapy* **36**, 657–663.

Prentice AG, Warnock DW, Johnson SA *et al.* (1994). Multiple dose pharmacokinetics of an oral solution of itraconazole in autologous bone marrow transplant recipients. *Journal of Antimicrobial Chemotherapy* **34**, 247–252.

Rex JH, Pfaller MA, Galgiani JN *et al.* (1997). Development of interpretive breakpoints for antifungal susceptibility testing: conceptual framework and analysis of *in vitro–in vivo* correlation data for fluconazole, itraconazole, and *Candida* infections. Subcommittee on Antifungal Susceptibility Testing of the National Committee for Clinical Laboratory Standards. *Clinical Infectious Diseases* **24**, 235–247.

Rogers TR (2001). Laboratory diagnosis of invasive fungal infections: impact of *in-vitro* tests on clinical management. In *The Effective Prevention and Management of Systemic Fungal Infection in Haematological Malignancy* (eds Prentice A, Rogers T and Miles A), pp. 41–47. Aesculapius Medical Press, London, UK.

Rosenberg-Arska M, Dekker AW, Branger J *et al.* (1991). A randomised study to compare oral fluconazole to amphotericin B in the prevention of fungal infections in patients with acute leukaemia. *Journal of Antimicrobial Chemotherapy* **27**, 369–376.

Slavin MA, Osborne B, Adams R *et al.* (1995). Efficacy and safety of fluconazole prophylaxis for fungal infections after marrow transplantation – a prospective, randomised, double blind study. *Journal of Infectious Diseases* **171**, 1545–1552.

Sugar AM (1993). Fluconazole and itraconazole: current status and prospects for anti-fungal therapy. *Current Clinical Topical Infectious Diseases* **13**, 74–98.

Tollemar J, Ringdon O, Andersson RS *et al.* (1993). Randomised double-blind study of liposomal amphoteracin B (AmBisome) prophylaxis of invasive fungal infections in bone marrow transplant recipients. *Bone Marrow Transplantation* **12**, 577–582.

Van Cutsem J, Van Gerven F, Janssen PAJ (1987). Activity of orally, topically, and parenterally administered itraconazole in the treatment of superficial and deep mycoses. *Reviews in Infectious Diseases* **9** (Suppl.1), S15–S32.

Vreugdenhil G, Van Dijke BJ, Donnelly JP *et al.* (1993). Efficacy of itraconazole in the prevention of fungal infections among neutropenic patients with haematologic malignancies and intensive chemotherapy. A double blind, placebo controlled study. *Leukaemia and Lymphoma* **11**, 353–358.

Walsh TJ, Finberg RW, Arndt C *et al.* (1999) for the National Institute of Allergy and Infectious Diseases Mycoses Study Group. Liposomal amphotericin B for empirical therapy in patients with persistent fever and neutropenia. *New England Journal of Medicine* **10**, 764–771.

Walsh TJ, Pappas PM, Winston DJ *et al.* (2002). Voriconazole compared with liposomal amphotericin B for empirical antifungal therapy in patients with neutropenia and persistent fever. *New England Journal of Medicine* **346**, 225–234.

Winston DJ, Maziarz RT, Chandrasekar PH *et al.* (2002). Long-term antifungal prophylaxis in allogeneic bone marrow transplant patients: A multicenter, randomised trial of intravenous/oral itraconazole versus fluconazole. *Blood* **98** (Suppl 1), 479a.

Chapter 6

Antifungal prophylaxis in the immunocompromised critically ill patient: an intensivist's perspective

Rick Keays

Introduction

The premise behind any form of prophylaxis is that there is a certainty that something will happen, or that there is a high likelihood that it will happen but you will know about it too late, and that it is undesirable. Deep fungal infection can be life threatening and is highly likely to occur in certain groups of patients, but our diagnostic facility prevents us from playing the waiting game. The rationale for antifungal prophylaxis for certain selected groups of critically ill patients has gathered momentum over the past few years. The trials that have been done show impressive results for reducing infection rates, but are too small to draw definitive conclusions about the ultimate goal of such a strategy: improved survival. The difficulty in limiting this chapter to a discussion of patients with neutropenia is that such patients rarely appear in the intensive care unit and most are encountered by physicians treating haematological malignancies where antifungal prophylaxis has an unchallenged role in management—or does it? I will examine some of the evidence that may undermine this role and also the evidence surrounding antifungal prophylaxis in those with immune compromise, notably HIV infection, post-transplantation and, of course, the critically ill.

Haematology

Neutropenia is commonly encountered by haematologists and rarely by intensivists. Neutropenic haematology patients are admitted to the intensive care unit—commonly for respiratory failure and/or sepsis. Survival is possible but the numbers are discouragingly low, especially if more than one organ system is failing (Brunet *et al.* 1990). Therefore the examination of antifungal prophylaxis in the neutropenic patient inevitably has to take account of the experience in haematology/oncology patients at an earlier stage. This article will address a personal interpretation of the literature in such patients and our experience of prophylaxis in the non-haematological patients.

Incidence

Neutropenic patients are vulnerable to infection; ergo they must be vulnerable to fungal infection. It has long been accepted that the lower the white cell count the greater the incidence of *Candida* antigenemia (Fanci *et al.* 1984). A single centre experience of fungal infection since 1980 reports that before 1991 the incidence was 1.8% of high-risk patients. From 1991 until 1993 there was a dramatic increase in incidence to 12% (De Laurenzi *et al.* 1996). This is at the lower end of estimates for the increase in systemic fungal infection rates. It is generally accepted that there has been a 10- to 20–fold increase over the past two decades.

Why has there been this apparent epidemic? Oral, gastrointestinal and systemic candidosis seem to be closely linked and oropharyngeal candidosis is very frequent. Predisposing factors such as damaged mucosal barriers due to chemotherapy, protracted periods of neutropenia, and prolonged use of antibiotics and steroids will inevitably increase the risk of deep mycoses. In a retrospective study of 73 patients with candidaemia, 26 patients died, of whom 19 died of *Candida* infection (Pagano *et al.* 1999). At univariate analysis colonisation, neutropenia, central venous lines and glycopeptide use was associated with an increased risk of candidaemia—interestingly, so was the use of antifungal prophylaxis.

Rationale

But what of prophylaxis? If the rationale for fungal chemoprophylaxis is the high incidence of fungal disease in these patients, the high mortality, the difficulty in diagnosing and the side effects of treatment (Amphotericin B), would it be useful—as opposed to empiric or directed treatment of the patient once they became febrile? Undoubtedly, fungemia in a neutropenic haematology patient is associated with a higher mortality than fungemia associated with other underlying disease states (Costa *et al.* 2000).

First suggestions that antifungals may help in neutropenic patients were well received; however, most of the trials compared one oral antifungal with another and involved few patients (Donnelly *et al.* 1984; Jones *et al.* 1984). Some concerns were raised that chemoprophylaxis may subsequently hamper the effect of full antifungal treatment when prophylaxis had failed (Schaffner & Frick 1985). Nevertheless oral antifungals remained a recommended therapy in neutropenic patients (Mayer & DeTorres 1985).

Pro

Somewhat tenuous support for prophylaxis came when two groups of neutropenic patients were compared, where one group had antibacterial *and* antifungal prophylaxis from the start and the other group had a treatment schedule that initiated once fever developed. Prophylaxis delayed the onset of a febrile illness but did not prevent positive fungal isolates. In the non-prophylaxis arm a patient died of *C. parakrusei* septicaemia (Schaison *et al.* 1990). However, the treatment protocols were complicated and the non-prophylaxis arm only received anti-fungals if fever relapsed while on antibacterial therapy, which may be viewed as too late.

More recent work on patients with acute leukaemia where the prophylaxis group was compared with historical controls has suggested a reduced mortality from proven fungal infection from 8.8% to 0.9% (Glasmacher *et al.* 1998). De Laurenzi *et al.* (1996) noted a dramatic reduction in incidence of fungal infection from 12% to 0.9% when oral, nasal and intravenous amphotericin B prophylaxis became part of the treatment policy. The GIMEMA Infection Program trial did demonstrate a clear difference in candidal infection rates when itraconazole prophylaxis was used, but *Aspergillus* infection was unaffected (Menichetti *et al.* 1999). Evidence supporting the long-term (75 days) use of fluconazole in blood and marrow transplant recipients noted a highly significant improved survival after an 8-year follow up. The incidence of invasive *Candida* infection was reduced from 20% to 2.6% (Marr *et al.* 2000).

An early paper that considered antifungal prophylaxis suggested that as there were no cases clinically identified as fungaemia then prophylaxis works. However, there was no placebo arm and one third of the patients autopsied (7/21) had evidence of fungal infection—mostly pulmonary aspergillosis (Meunier-Carpentier *et al.* 1983). After 1990 this problem of inverse logic is seen to be applied again. Clinical ignorance of a problem does not mean it isn't there—as the autopsy evidence reveals. As recently as 2000 the following statement was made in a paper from the USA looking at marrow transplant recipients: 'In this prospective trial, low-dose amphotericin B prophylaxis was as effective as fluconazole prophylaxis.' (Wolff *et al.* 2000). But one could substitute 'effective' for 'ineffective' with a transformation in the conclusion but no loss of sense. Indeed the incidence of proven fungal infection was 5.6% in the group as a whole, which may be viewed as lower than expected—or it might not.

In a trial of nystatin versus fluconazole prophylaxis for leukaemia patients undergoing chemotherapy, there appeared to be significant reduction in unexplained febrile episodes with fluconazole but no statistical difference in systemic fungal infection rates. 'Prophylaxis was successful (no evidence of fungal infection or fever of unknown origin unresponsive to antibiotics) in 38 of 56 (68%) fluconazole-treated and 25 of 53 (47%) nystatin-treated patients (p = 0.03). 2 patients (4%) in the fluconazole group and 6 (11%) patients in the nystatin group developed systemic fungal infections (p = 0.15).' The authors concluded that fluconazole was more effective at preventing candidaemia (Young *et al.* 1999).

There appears to be an element of wishful thinking in the interpretation of results. Autopsy evidence was used to determine whether invasive fungal infection was present in a paediatric population, comparing the period before a prophylaxis protocol was instituted and thereafter. The incidence of invasive infections was the same but the authors concluded that chemotherapy régimes had become more aggressive over time so a lack of expected rise in infection rates was proof of prophylaxis efficacy—which is hardly cast-iron evidence (Kato *et al.* 1995). And what evidence there is is often indirect: a study of solid tumour and haematology patients with proven fungal infection demonstrated that mortality independently correlated with a lack of prior antifungal prophylaxis (Viscoli *et al.* 1999).

There is also some confusion about what is prophylaxis and what is treatment. One randomised controlled trial (RCT) with fairly large numbers of patients comparing miconazole with placebo actually meant starting when a fever was apparent, which is hardly prophylaxis. However, it did show significantly reduced rates of both non-fatal and fatal fungal infections (Wingard *et al.* 1987).

Con

A study from Germany examining fluconazole prophylaxis looked at 68 patients with acute myelocytic leukaemia (AML) and came to the opposite conclusion. There was neither a reduction in fever of unknown origin nor of invasive fungal infection in the prophylaxis group (Kern *et al.* 1998). This was also emphasised in another large study where fluconazole prophylaxis was compared with placebo during episodes of chemotherapy-induced neutropenia. Empiric use of amphotericin B was delayed in the fluconazole group but systemic infection rates were not reduced (Schaffner & Schaffner 1995). The healthcare costs were not reduced either in the fluconazole group. Most well-conducted trials have failed to show a significant reduction in systemic fungal infection rates or mortality (Vreugdenhil *et al.* 1993; Winston *et al.* 1993).

A review of 355 autopsies performed on patients who had undergone bone marrow transplantation (BMT) looked at the effect of fluconazole prophylaxis on the presence of fungal infection. There was no difference in fungal infection rates with or without fluconazole. However, *Aspergillus* infection was noted in 29% of patients who has received fluconazole compared with only 18% of those who had not. The authors speculated that the decline in *Candida* infections due to fluconazole allowed the patients to survive longer and thus contract *Aspergillus* infection (van Burik *et al.* 1998).

Pathogen shift

Antifungals can reduce colonisation rates (de Vries-Hospers *et al.* 1982) but have a tendency to favour emergence of less sensitive organisms. An old paper, comparing ketoconazole with nystatin orally, showed that colonisation rates were around 26–47% but fungal sepsis only occurred in 2/56 patients (Shepp *et al.* 1985). A tendency to shift to *C. glabrata* was noted. Several subsequent studies have confirmed that the consequence of widespread use of antifungals leads to resistance. This tendency for pathogen shift is a worrying consequence of prophylaxis (Boogaerts *et al.* 1989; Krcmery *et al.* 1999). Over time pathogen shift is inevitable and the hospital becomes the reservoir for such relatively resistant organisms (Salonen *et al.* 2000).

Conclusion

There is a problem. Fungal infection rates have increased 20–fold in the past two decades in these patients while antifungal prophylaxis has also been increasing. So it is either a genuine increase due to changes in patient management, or prophylaxis is not working, or detection rates have improved. This problem has surely been created by the antimicrobial policies that have been accepted practice. Empirical broad spectrum antibiotic poly-pharmacy has undoubtedly contributed to the huge increase in invasive yeast and mould infections. This approach has caused a disastrous shift towards resistant bacterial and increasing fungal infection rates (Maertens & Boogaerts 1998). Recent efforts have been to rein in this approach and aim for guided antibacterial monotherapy, or at least patient-tailored rather than protocol-driven therapy.

So what do the experts think of antifungal prophylaxis? Antifungal prophylaxis of candidosis with both non- and absorbable drugs was not convincing for reduction of proven fungal infections (Hoffken 1989). This situation still pertains over a decade later: 'Antifungal prophylaxis has been effective in reducing candida infection, however, there has been no proven successful prevention of invasive aspergillosis. In addition, there is no clearly proven benefit of antifungal prophylaxis regarding the reduction in the overall mortality. Thus the best way to reduce invasive fungal-related mortality will be early diagnosis and pre-emptive therapeutic approaches.' (Bohme *et al.* 1999). A clear desire exists for better diagnosis by using imaging techniques such as the high-resolution computerised tomography (CT) scan and new methods for detecting fungi such as *Aspergillus* galactomannan, so that it may be possible to move away from prophylaxis towards pre-emptive treatment (Donnelly 2000). However, formal clinical trials will be needed to clarify this approach.

Prophylaxis does work to reduce colonisation rates and it seems to reduce dissemination rates (Ellis *et al.* 1994). But it is still unclear whether prophylaxis or earlier pre emptive treatment is the best policy to adopt. Indeed, most of the studies looking at fluconazole as a prophylactic agent use a dose of 400 mg/day, which is actually a treatment dose for *C. albicans* and inadequate for other organisms. The literature is confused and is not helped by the recent Cochrane Collaboration meta-analysis that came to the conclusion that antifungal prophylaxis is of no benefit (Gotzsche & Johansen 2000). What is true is that prophylaxis may falsely reassure the physician—drug levels may be inadequate in preventing infection. The concern that non-*albicans* species may make an appearance is a real and significant danger. Itraconazole may be the best prophylaxis of the currently available azoles in that it has activity against *Aspergillus*, which in many units is as much of a problem than *Candida* (Morgenstern *et al.* 1999), but it has unpredictable absorption and levels may need to be monitored. The solution is better than the capsules and an intravenous preparation is now available but should probably be reserved for empiric treatment.

Other measures perhaps need to be emphasised. *Aspergillus* infection rates have been reduced by controlling the environment of the patient during the period of neutropenia with high-efficiency particulate air filtering (Withington *et al.* 1998). Probiosis may be helpful, as a paper from over 20 years ago has suggested in a pediatric population of neutropenic patients. Framycetin, colymycin, nystatin and metronidazole gut decontamination were compared with cotrimoxazole and lactobacilli preparations (Ekert *et al.* 1980). There was no difference in infection rates between the two groups and the latter prophylaxis was much better tolerated—possibly the lactobacilli were the key?

AIDS and antifungal prophylaxis

The prognosis for patients with AIDS admitted to the intensive care unit was initially dire and then improved in the late 1980s and early 1990s. There has subsequently been an ever-worsening outlook. This can be explained by improvements in anti-retroviral therapy and *Pneumocystis carinii* pneumonia (PCP) prophylaxis such that fewer patients are now admitted but at a more advanced and therapeutically resistant stage of disease. In the 4 years from 1997 in our unit, which is the largest HIV treatment centre in the UK, the ITU mortality was 68% and the in-hospital mortality was 85%. Antifungal prophylaxis is not the issue by the time such individuals are admitted to the intensive-care unit.

Nevertheless, there is a cogent case for antifungal prophylaxis before such deterioration. There has been an increase in the fungal infection rates in HIV-positive individuals because of the inherent immunological susceptibility and the increasing incidence of neutropenia coupled with use of steroids. The risk of infection is approximately the same as the normal population if the CD4 count is maintained above 400/mm^3. Below this level *Candida* and *Cryptococcus* are the main infective organisms but *Aspergillus* is on the increase. Most cases of histoplasmosis, coccidioidomycosis and blastomycosis occur in regions where their causative organisms are endemic (Ampel 1996). *Penicillium marneffei* infection is very common in HIV-infected individuals in Asia.

Prophylaxis in this group of patients represents one of the greatest challenges and risks to the currently available therapeutic armamentarium. Because it is often required for exceptionally long periods of time with limited prospect for immunological improvement, the chances of prophylaxis failure, resistance and deleterious changes to the mycoflora are at their highest.

The incidence of oral *Candida* colonisation in HIV-positive individuals is high (around 85%) and does not seem to be influenced by the use of antifungal prophylaxis (Schmidt-Westhausen *et al.* 1991). The susceptibility to fungal infection is evident and the use of both prophylaxis and actual treatment for the distressing symptoms of mucocutaneous infection has made the use of antifungals in this group widespread. Not surprisingly, this has led to the emergence of resistance. The first